Crisis Prevention

Subclinical Signs of Impending Doom

Carol Whiteside, RN, PhD

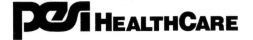

Continuing Education Self Study Credit Available: PESI HealthCare
provides self study credit for this publication. Please see the information
contained in the back of this book for details.

**For information on this and other PESI HealthCare products, please
call 800-843-7763**

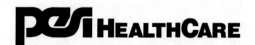

www.pesihealthcare.com

About the Author

C arol Whiteside RN, Ph.D.(c) graduated from Baylor University School of Nursing, Dallas, Texas in 1972. Her nursing experience includes adult, pediatric, and newborn ICUs, adult and pediatric open heart, burn and trauma units, cath labs, and clinical education. She is a nurse entrepreneur presenting courses in critical care topics, EKG interpretation, ACLS, critical thinking, and a variety of other nursing topics, teaching at her local nursing schools, and traveling for PESIHealthCare. Carol is graduate of the Cardiovascular Nurse Specialist program at The Methodist Hospital, Texas Medical Center in Houston. She received her Masters in Nursing and PhD from Gonzaga University. Her dissertation was the Leadership of Florence Nightingale.

Table of Contents

Introduction

Human physiology is like a finely choreographed ballet. It is gentle and it is fierce. It is logical and it is obedient. If everything performs as it should, there is health. If an event does not obey the rules (pathophysiology), there is dysfunction and illness. All we have to do is figure what the rules are. The problem with the rules is that our understanding of them keeps changing as our knowledge of how the body works increases.

At any given moment in time, our knowledge and actions have a 50% error rate. Fifty percent of what you are doing at work is wrong. The trouble is, we don't know which 50% it is! We do things because they look like a really good idea until further research shows it wasn't such a good idea and we stop doing it. We used to administer lidocaine IV drips on patients with a diagnosis of "rule out MI," or give aminophyline drips to everyone who wheezed once in the emergency room. Both of these treatments were shown to increase complications and death, and neither are practiced today.

We are working with the best information we have, but that information is constantly being updated, and we need to stay updated also. Changes are occurring faster today that at any other time in history and, they show no sign of slowing down. Nurses care for patients with higher acuity rates than ever before, and nurses are expected to know more than ever before. The nurse's job is not one of crisis *management*, it is one of crisis *prevention*.

To prevent a crisis, you must be able to see it coming before it arrives. *Clinical* signs are the ones they taught in nursing school: vital signs, lung sounds, neuro-vascular checks, etc. These signs are great for recognizing a dilemma because they occur *after* the body's compensatory mechanisms have failed to correct the problem. What if we could see the signs that compensation was taking place *before* the process failed? We can. It is these *subclinical* signs of impending doom that this book will depict—how to tell your patients are going bad before they keel over and die.

Everything—every thought, every movement, every action in the body—has a physiologic, and therefore chemical basis. The smallest living units in the body are its cells. The action and events occurring on a cellular level are those that spell wellness or illness in the human body. It is imperative that we understand some cellular metabolism in order to understand those compensatory mechanisms that we want to observe.

The Cell and the City

1

The first thing you need to do is to have what is called a paradigm shift. By that, I mean that you need to stop thinking about things in one way and start thinking about them in another way. You need to stop thinking about your patients as *macro* individuals and start thinking about them as very large collections of microscopic cells. You must understand that every single cell in the human body is a living, breathing entity on its own. When you die, you die one cell at a time. When you save someone's life, you do it one cell at a time. The more cells that you have living, the more likely you are to have a living patient.

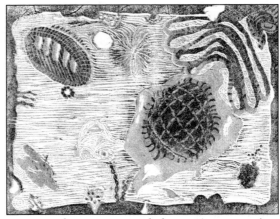

All cells possess the same needs, wants, and dynamics as a city. Every cell in the body has to have and be able to do everything that a city has to have and be able to do.

POWER

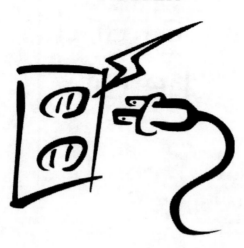

POWER IN THE CITY

A city must have a source of power. No power, no city. The more sources and quantity of power there is, the bigger the city gets to be. We use power to heat our homes, run farm machinery, manufacture, transportation, cook our food, and countless other things which could not occur without power. If we had no source of power, we would be back in the stone age at a time before the discovery of fire.

POWER IN THE CELL

Inside the cell there must be a source of power. For the human body there is one source of power—Adenosinetriphosphate, or ATP. If you fire a neuron, you use ATP. If you contract a muscle, you use ATP. If you make a new red blood cell, you use ATP. It is the only energy source in your body. ATP is made in the cell in a structure called the mitochondria. The number of mitochondria you find in a cell is directly proportional to the amount of energy that cell needs to produce. For example, hummingbird muscles have 10 times more mitochondria that the average bird wing muscle has. Cardiac cells have more mitochondria than skeletal muscle cells because they work continuously.

WATER

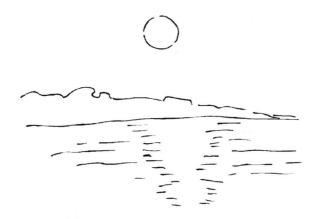

WATER IN THE CITY

A city must be near a source of water. No water, no city. The larger the source of water, the bigger the city can become. You do all kinds of things with water in the city; you drink it, you wash things it in, you cook with it, you float things on it for commerce, and you splash in it to cool off. Every city has a source of water and the city depends on its continued presence for its existence.

WATER IN THE CELL

In the body there are several places for water to be: inside the cell (intracellular), outside the cell (extracellular), and in the vascular space within the blood vessels. Maintaining the proper amount of fluid in these spaces is crucial for the life of the macro individual. Fluid is so crucial that if the volume and thereby the pressure is dropping off in the vascular space, the body will draw from the extracellular space to fill the vascular space back up. Then as the extracellular volume and thereby the pressure drops off, the body will draw fluid from the intracellular space to refill the extracellular space. Patients so severely dehydrated that they have sunken in eyeballs have depleted all three spaces. By the same token, if the volume and thereby the pressure increases in the vascular space, fluid is forced into the extracellular space where it is called edema. This is the mechanism for ankle edema, ascites, pulmonary edema, etc.

As the extracellular volume increases, it will force fluid into the intracellular space. Having the right amount of fluid in the right spaces is crucial to the life of the *macro* individual due to the inner workings of the *micro* individual, or the cell.

Where to find water in the body:

- Intracellular space
- Extracellular space
- Vascular space within the blood vessels

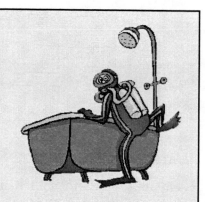

Inside the cell there are all kinds of little organelles and structures that make the cell work. If the cell is dehydrated, these structures are all shrunken in on themselves, and they don't work right. If the cell is overhydrated, these structures get pulled apart, and again, they don't work right. The proper functioning of the cell requires proper fluid volumes in all spaces.

Your body is equipped with all kinds of sensors monitoring how things are going in the body. One set of these sensors are called *osmoreceptors*. They look at the *osmolality*—the concentration or dilution—of your blood. The osmoreceptors are tied directly into your thirst mechanism. If your blood is becoming concentrated, you *will* go get something to drink. Have you ever noticed how much patients *hate* being placed on fluid restrictions? Patients placed on fluid restrictions have been known to drink from the toilet. Imagine how strong an urge someone would have to have for her to take a cup from the kitchen, go down the hall to the bathroom, scoop water out of the toilet, and drink it down.

That's how strong your thirst mechanism is. You will drink from the toilet before you will allow yourself to die of thirst. If you put someone on a fluid restriction, you are asking him to go against what is probably his second most basic drive. The body's most basic drive is the drive to take a breath; the second is to balance the body's fluids. Balancing fluids is essential to the functioning of the cells and therefore is essential to life.

FOOD

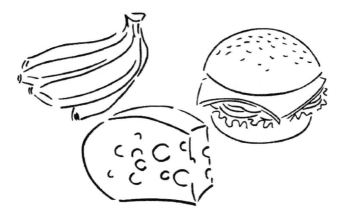

FOOD IN THE CITY

It is easy to buy pineapples, wheat, or rice in the city, but chances are the are grown outside the city. That means there needs to be an intricate system of importing and exporting to get all the things needed for the city. Open lines of transportation and vehicles of some type are required. If the city's means of importing should break down, the city's vitality would be seriously curtailed.

FOOD IN THE CELL

The cell also needs food. Have you ever wondered what you do with the food you eat? Before you store it on your hips, there are three crucial things you do with it: you make energy from it, you repair your infrastructure, and you "make stuff" out of it.

Right now your body is making epinephrine. It is making red blood cells. It is making all kinds of things from the food you eat. If you didn't eat it, inhale it, or absorb it through your skin, it isn't a part of your body.

When your body makes a new red blood cell, it lasts about 120 days. A neutrophil lasts only 24 hours, so every 24 hours you have to make new neutrophils. If your patient has an albumin of less that 1.5, he physiologically lacks the building blocks (biological substrates) to make a scar. You must give your patients the building blocks to make things like an active immune system or a normal hemoglobin, and these building blocks are called food.

Feeding our patients is not easy. Many patients challenge our ability to be creative, but you can't just *not* feed them. They can't heal themselves if you don't give them the building blocks to do it with. Use your clinical dietitian to find some way to get nutrients into the patient.

Getting the biological substrates that have been eaten out to the cells requires an intact circulatory system. Have you ever had a patient with a non-healing ulcer on his foot who was sent away for an arteriogram? You may have been thinking, *"What's he going for an arteriogram for? What he needs is an antibiotic."* But if there isn't an intact circulatory system into the ulcer, there's no way to get the antibiotic down to it. You must eat the biological substrates, but you must also have an intact circulatory system to get it out to where it needs to be used. If you can't improve the blood flow, amputations are often required.

There is a system of selectivity in the cells. If you want a substance to have an effect inside a cell, you must have a gate or receptor site for that substance. This makes good sense. You can't have every cell in the body being affected by every chemical or hormone in the bloodstream. If you want Angiotensin II to have an effect, you must have an Angiotensin II receptor site. Otherwise, it will just float on by.

These receptor site are very dynamic. For example, should you block one of the receptors with a beta blocking agent (a beta blocker blocks beta receptors on the cell membrane), the cell will respond to the lack of expected input by up-regulating the number of beta receptors on the cell membrane. The beta blocker dose must then be increased to block the new receptors. For this reason, patients must never abruptly stop taking beta blockers. They must be weaned off their beta blockers to allow the cells to down regulate receptors on the cell membrane.

We have also learned that you up- and down-regulate these receptors from the cell membrane based on your circadian rhythms. The chemicals floating around in your blood stream affect you differently at different parts of the day. (This is another reason why night shift is so physically and mentally difficult for most of us.)

One substance cells require most often is glucose. Cells use glucose to make energy. If your patient has a blood sugar of 450, his energy level is terrible. This is an indication that the glucose is not in the cells but out in the blood stream. What do you give a patient to drive glucose into the cell? Insulin is a marvelous hormone that does lots of things in the body, but one thing it will do is bind to the glucose in the circulatory system. On the cell membrane, there is a gate. Insulin holds the key to that gate. It binds to the glucose, opens the gate, brings the glucose into the cell, drops it off where the mitochondria can make ATP out of it, and up goes your patient's energy level. A patient with a blood glucose of 450 and one with a blood glucose of 25 can have the same pathetic energy level because glucose is not getting into their cells. Glucose must be inside the cells or it might as well not be there at all.

WE DON'T KNOW WHAT WE ARE DOING

We want the best for our patients. Unfortunately, we don't always know what we are doing. At any given moment in time, half of what we are doing is wrong. The only problem is that we don't know which half it is. What this means is that we have to stay current on the latest research, and in medicine, new research means things change constantly.

I think the term *diabetes* is a good example of how we don't always know what we are doing. When I got out of nursing school in the early 70s, I knew what a diabetic was. There were two kinds: adult and juvenile. But then some adults started getting juvenile diabetes, and some of the juveniles started getting the adult form. So we decided to call the two forms *insulin dependent* and *non-insulin dependent* diabetes. But then some non-insulin dependent diabetics became insulin dependent, and then became non-insulin dependent again. So we gave them nice, non-descriptive terms: Type I and Type II. But now we have another problem. What about the patients called *insulin resistant* or *glucose intolerant?* Are we looking at the possibility of a *Type III* diabetes? Type I is a failure to produce insulin; Type II is a problem with the gate; Type III may become a problem with the key. The knowledge base of medicine is constantly in flux, and we must stay informed on the latest research. We don't know anything for certain, except that we all got born somehow and eventually we all die.

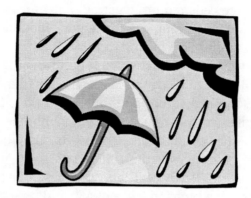

STORM DRAINAGE SYSTEMS IN THE CITY

From time to time it rains too much in the city, so they have storm drainage systems to carry the water out of the city to the river where it goes back into the ecosystem. Without this protective device, cities would stay wet much longer and have more damage from flooding.

STORM DRAINAGE SYSTEM IN THE CELL

The body's storm drainage system is called the *lymph* system. We are constantly producing too much fluid around our cells, but it's never a problem because the fluid is picked up by the lymph system, dumped back into the central venous system, and recycled. On a good day, this works very well for us.

There is, however, another fluid problem in the cell that requires a very specialized sump system. Ions flux in and out of the cells all the time for many different reasons. One ion that comes in a lot is Calcium. This wouldn't be a problem except that frequently when Ca + + comes in it is holding the hand of its friend Na + . This also wouldn't be a problem, except that most Na + ions have seven water molecules attached to them. If all this sodium and water were allowed to stay inside the cells they would swell up and burst.

To fix this problem, on the walls of every single cell in your body you have a Na+ – K+ – ATP pump to remove all that sodium and water. This is the largest use of energy in your body.

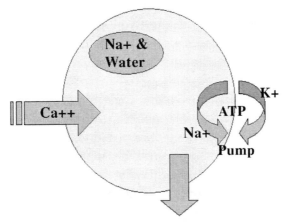

Na+ and water back out

As soon as your patient stops making ATP in sufficient amounts, every single cell in the body begins to swell up, and if left unchecked, the cells will eventually burst. This swelling and eventual lysing is the mechanism for necrosis, and as you well know, once something has necrotized, it's never coming back again.

When you save someone's life, you do it one cell at a time. You die one cell at a time, and you save someone's life one cell at a time. The very first thing that you have to do to save someone's life is to keep those Na+ – K+ – ATP pumps running. The way you do that is by oxygenating and perfusing *at the same time*. You cannot do one at expense of the other. They must be simultaneous. As soon as oxygenation or perfusion is neglected the cells begin to swell, become dysfunctional and eventually undergo lysis, never to return again.

If a young, healthy patient is in shock, you may feel that if you can just get some fluid and drugs going, you should be able to save him. You may be surprised when this patient dies anyway. It all has to do with the total number of cells left alive at the end of the untoward event, whether or not oxygenation and perfusion were maintained.

One night, a group of young men were driving around in a car with a gun. They were playing around with the gun when it discharged and blew apart one kid's femoral artery. At this point, all the kids in the car panicked. They were not supposed to be together, much less in a car with a gun, so they continued to drive around for a while trying to decide what to do while the victim bled out. By the time they realized they had a problem that they couldn't deal with, they had stopped at a rest stop on the interstate, which put them even further from help.

When the paramedics got there, they pulled the young man out of the car, started CPR, and got some lines and fluid into him. The paramedics said there were five inches of blood on the floor of the car. They brought the young man into the ED, where they worked on him for about an hour and a half. Eventually they got some semblance of a heartbeat and blood pressure back. At that point he was sent to surgery to have his femoral artery repaired. Since no one dies in surgery, he officially died in PACU. He went into Disseminated Intravascular Coagulaopathy (DIC), used up all his clotting factors making microscopic clots, and bled to death. This young man had so much cellular death before the paramedics even arrived that there was truly nothing to get back. If you ever save the life of a patient who has marginally enough cells left to be alive, they are usually so severely damaged that you may wish you had never begun resuscitation.

> # OXYGENATE & PERFUSE
> ## AT THE SAME TIME
> ## WITHOUT EXCEPTION!

To save someone's life, you must oxygenate and perfuse at the same time. You must keep those $Na+ - K+ - ATP$ pumps running. If the patient is breathing and oxygenating well, you don't have to do a thing. If not, you step in immediately and breathe for them. If there is a good heart rate and blood pressure, nothing is required from you. If there isn't, you step in immediately and get that heart rate and blood pressure adequate or the cells will begin to lyse. The more cells you have alive, the more likely you are to get a living patient.

SANITATION IN THE CITY

If there was no sanitation in your city how long could your city exist? Probably not too long. In a city there are different kinds of waste being produced requiring different kinds of waste removal. There's human excrement, grass clippings, recyclable things, and hazardous waste from the hospitals, among other things. Each of these requires its own waste management program so as not to harm the city.

SANITATION IN THE CELLS

The same system is in the body. There are different kinds of waste being produced and different kinds of waste removal systems available. The kidneys, lungs, GI tract, and skin get rid of waste for us. When you have a chemical reaction inside a cell, you sometimes produce a toxic by-product. If you have another chemical reaction, and right away change the toxin into something that is not toxic, we say you buffered it. That is your intracellular buffer system.

But sometimes you produce substances that are so toxic you can't buffer them. For these you will need a specialized kind of waste removal system, and your body has one. It's called a lysome. The lysome is an organelle within in the cell. You take your extremely toxic substance and you encapsulate it—you can't have it damaging the inner workings of the cell. You move it over to the lysome and dump it

13

in. The lysome has extremely caustic enzymes in it, and it will get rid of this nasty substance for you. That's the good part. The bad part is that it has extremely caustic enzymes in it and it is sitting right in the middle of the cell. If the lysome's membrane should break down, the cell dies. And as this dead cell's wall breaks down, the caustic enzymes come up against the wall of the cell next door. The result is a cascading cellular death, which is not good for a long and healthy life.

What can cause lysomal membranes to break down? First, if a cell swells up because the $N+ - K+ - ATP$ pumps are not kept running by adequate oxygenation and perfusion, the lysome will be pulled apart. The inflammatory process can also cause lysomal membranes to break down, which, in turn, can cause the death of your patient. Prednisone is a drug that stabilizes lysomal membranes in the face of inflammation so that when you are done with your untoward event, you have more cells alive that you have dead, and that's a good thing. So we will oxygenate and perfuse at the same time to prevent cellular swelling and use prednisone in the face of inflammation.

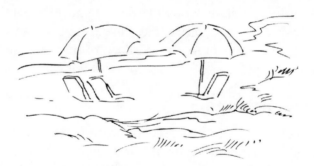

THE CITY AND ENVIRONMENT

The location of any city is dependent on the environment. If a city can respond and adapt to the environment, it thrives. If it can't, it dies. In cold environments, houses have heating systems. In hot environments they have air conditioners. When Ann Bancroft and Liv Arnesen trekked across the Antarctic continent, they didn't meet anyone. It is entirely too hard to respond and adapt to that environment for any human settlement to become established and thrive.

THE CELL AND ENVIRONMENT

The cells in your body also have an optimal environment determined by the pH. The pH in your body needs to be 7.35 to 7.45—*period.* If the pH increases or decreases to an amount outside this range, every single cell in the body becomes dysfunctional. Get far enough outside this range and the cells begin to die off. You cannot walk around with your pH out of alignment.

The human body does a great job responding and adapting to the environment. CO_2 retaining COPDers become acidotic, but they retain bicarb and swing their pH back to normal. People in renal failure walk around with a BUN and Creatinine so high most of us couldn't stand up with it. People with chronic anemia are out walking around with a Hg/Hct most of us couldn't sit on the side of the bed with. If change happens slowly, the body does a wonderful job of responding and adapting. If it happens fast, the body may be in trouble. They say that what doesn't kill us makes us stronger, and that does appear to be true.

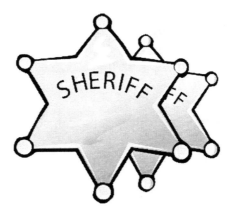

THE CITY, BOSSES AND RULES

A city needs a boss—someone to set the rules and keep law and order. Law and order is important so that the city can keep on with its day to day business. Would you have left home to go to work or school if you thought there was a pretty good chance that your house would be ransacked, burned to the ground, and your children kidnapped while you were gone? (Does it depend on how your kids acted at breakfast that morning?) The reason you don't have to camp out in the front yard with a shotgun is because we have rules that society follows. Usually.

THE CELL, BOSSES AND RULES

Inside the cell, you need a boss. There is only one boss inside the cell and that is the DNA. DNA runs everything. DNA is so important to the cell that it is encapsulated in its own nuclear membrane to protect it from the inner workings of the cell. If you should damage your DNA—and we do from time to time—the cell takes a look at the DNA that comes before and after the break and tries to replicate the damaged part.

The rules for governing your body are strict. The rules are called *homeostasis*—the body's own equilibrium. Your body is a fascist organization. There is no free thinking allowed among the cells. Each cell will do the job it is born to do, never think about another job, and work as hard as it can. When the cell can no longer put out at 100% effort, we kill it off and get a nice new cell to take its place.

We are happy because of this. We can't have pulmonary cells that decide they would like to be cardiac cells for a while. We can't have chemical messengers that decide that they will take a mental health day. We can't have cells that decide they want to spike their hair and pierce their noses. When cells do that they are called cancer cells.

Your body is making cancer cells right now. But instead of gathering them into little groups and rehabilitating them, your body is killing them off just as fast as it can. There is a cell in your immune system called a natural killer cell. This cell roams the body looking for cells that aren't with the program. He sides up next to it, inserts a tube, injects a poison, pulls out the tube, and goes on his merry way looking for the next errant cell. Remember, you make the natural cells, as well as the rest of your immune system, out of the food you eat. How important is nutrition in preventing cancer? How important is nutrition to cancer patients or any patient trying to fight off a disease or trauma? How much attention do we pay to it? We are getting better, but we still have a long way to go.

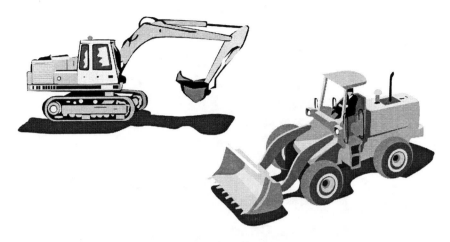

INFRASTRUCTURE REPAIR IN THE CITY

As much as you hate it when they tear up the roads in your city, you would hate it a lot more if they *never* tore up the roads. A city repairs the roads, sewers, electrical system, communication systems, and other infrastructure on a near-constant basis. Infrastructure repair is an ongoing project that consumes huge amounts of resources. When funds are tight, infrastructure repair is one of the first things to get cut back. If this goes on long enough, the city falls into disrepair, becomes dangerous, and may eventually die.

INFRASTRUCTURE REPAIR IN THE CELL

The same process is going on inside the cell and the body. We repair ourselves constantly. We repair our cell membranes, nuclear membranes, valve leaflets, gastric mucosa, skin, bones, and on and on. This repair is made with our reserve—what is left over.

Consider how quickly the human body decomposes. Up until the moment of death, the body puts that much time and effort into repairs. The problem with a lot of our patients is that they don't have any reserve with which to make repairs, and it is our job to give them that reserve, because they are the only ones who can make that repair.

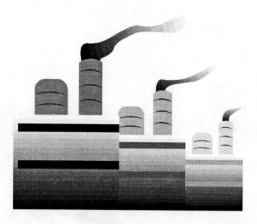

MANUFACTURING IN THE CITY

Earlier, I had said that a city requires a vigorous import and export system to get all it needs to function. That implies that there is something of value to pay for the imported stuff. If the city sits on top of a gold mine, all it needs do is chip off little pieces of gold to pay for things. But eventually the gold runs out. So the city may turn to other resources. It may cut down all the trees, kill off all the buffalo, or fish out all the lakes and rivers. With nothing left to trade, a city must turn to manufacturing.

If you are going to manufacture something, the most efficient way to do it is inside a factory with an assembly line. To make a car, the first thing you do is put down the wheels, then the engine, then the chassis, then the windows, and before long you've got a car. Because of this, it is going to be very important that things are in the right place on the assembly line. You can't have the windows at the beginning and the wheels at the end.

Things must be in the proper order, and if you are running out of any one thing—engines, for example—you will be done making completed cars until you get more. So, someone has to be looking at the supplies on the assembly line. If engines are running low, they go back to the well stocked warehouse, get more engines, put them in exactly the right spot on the assembly line, and go back and order more engines to restock the warehouse. It is a complex process designed to keep the assembly line humming along and productivity high.

MANUFACTURING IN THE CELLS

This is exactly the same process used by your cells to make things. They use an assembly line called the endoplasmic reticulum. Let's say we have a cell that is going to make insulin. It makes insulin based on blood sugar values among other things. Which means the cell knows what the blood sugar is. You don't want it cranking out insulin if the blood sugar is low. On the cell membrane there is a sensor receiving information about the blood sugar. It passes this information via a chemical messenger to the nucleus where the DNA resides.

The DNA decides whether or not to make insulin. The DNA never leaves the protection of the nucleus. It sends its messenger, the RNA, out into the cytoplasm to the endoplasmic reticulum to deliver the news. The messenger RNA goes out and says, "Alright, guys, kick it up, we're going to make some insulin and here is the blueprint on how the DNA wants it done." The RNA comes out with a blueprint of where to put which amino acids on the assembly line. Remember some cells make more than one substance, and this blueprint will change.

When you look at cells making things, remember there must always be a signal to turn the process on. We are pretty good at remembering that. Remember there must always be a signal to turn the process off. We are only fair at remembering that. But, what we are awful at remembering, is that you must get rid of what ever you made. How many gallons of epinephrine have you made in your life time? How many swimming pools of cerebral spinal fluid did you generate last year? How many trillion red blood cells have you made? Where has it all gone? You must turn the process on, turn the process off, *and* get rid of what ever it is you made. These are three areas where disease can occur and three areas where drugs can work.

Imagine that we are going to make insulin. First, there must be a signal to turn the process on. Insulin is a long chain amino acid. Amino acids must come from the food you eat. They are transported to the cell via an intact circulatory system. The cell lines the amino acids up along the endoplasmic reticulum and a signal turns the process on. As the molecule of insulin comes down the assembly line you add the first amino acid, then the second, then the third, etc, etc, until out the end comes a long chain amino acid called insulin.

After the insulin molecule is made, it is not automatically released into the blood stream. The body must have a reserve of insulin. The cell must decide whether to release the insulin into the blood stream or store it in the reserve to be used at another time.

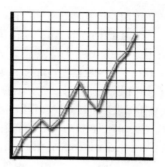

PRODUCTIVITY IN THE CITY

The name of the game is productivity, and to that end you need healthy, motivated workers in sufficient numbers to get the job done. Workers get days off from work for their health. They are supposed to rest so that they can repair their own infrastructures and be more productive when they come back to work. (You do rest on your days off, don't you?)

Motivation is crucial to productivity. Have you ever worked with someone who didn't share the group's common goal? Did that person harm the productivity of the group? Productivity greatly increases if we are all working together toward the same end.

If you have too many workers, you strain the resources. If you have too few workers, you can't get the job done. Having the right number of healthy, motivated workers will ensure good productivity.

PRODUCTIVITY IN THE CELL

The cell is also concerned with productivity—getting done whatever it is supposed to be doing. A healthy cell is one with plenty of biological substrates, a repaired infrastructure, and lots of ATP available. As for motivation, all the cells in your body share one common goal, and that is to keep you alive. To that end, you will see numerous compensatory mechanisms go into play to try and keep you alive before you are allowed to die.

It is the activation of some of these compensatory mechanisms that are the basis for the subclinical signs of impending doom. Have you ever been blind-sided by a catastrophic event with a patient and after the crisis was over and you had time to think, you wondered, "Could I, should I, have seen it coming?" There is a saying in radiology that states, "You only see what you know." What this means is that if you don't know something exists, you wouldn't be able to identify it even if it was staring you right in the face. The rest of this book dedicated to helping you recognize the signs that compensatory mechanisms have been activated. These signs are based in pathophysiology.

KEY INGREDIENTS FOR CHAPTER 1

1. When you die you do it one cell at a time.
2. When you save someone's life you do it one cell at a time.
3. To keep cells from swelling up and lysing, you need to keep the sodium – potassium – ATP pumps running. You do this by oxygenating and perfusing at the same time—not one at the expense of the other.
4. Protect the integrity of lysomal membranes by oxygenating and perfusing at the same time and using prednisone if there is an inflammatory process.
5. If you expect someone to heal they need the biological substrates to do it with and ATP will be the energy source

Energy and Purpose

2

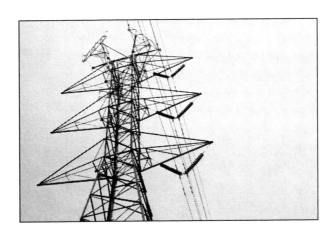

ADENOSINE TRIPHOSPHATE

L et's revisit our friend adenosine triphosphate (ATP), the only energy source in the body. You make ATP via a process called oxidative phosphorylation. Oxidative phosphorylation is the most efficient way your body has to take the food that you eat and turn it into energy. It does it in the walls of the mitochondria via the Kreb's Cycle. I do believe nurses were universally traumatized by the Kreb's Cycle in school. We do our very best to never think of it because it was such an disagreeable experience to see it appear on a test. What you clearly remember about the Kreb's Cycle, however, is that if you have both oxygen and glucose and throw it into the cycle, ATP comes out the other end. With both glucose and oxygen present, you get 37 ATP every time you run the cycle and you obviously run it zillions of times to meet the body's needs.

$$\text{Glucose} + \text{Oxygen} = 37 \text{ ATP}$$

Now, because your body wants to keep you alive, you can run the system without oxygen for a short period of time if you want to. If you run it anaerobically, however, you only get three ATP each time. How is your patient's energy level as soon as they become hypoxic? It decreases, doesn't it? And the amount it decreases is directly proportional to how hypoxic they become.

$$\text{Glucose} - \text{Oxygen} = 3 \text{ ATP} + \text{lactic acid}$$

Not only does the patient's energy level decrease, but they also begin to crank out lactic acid. The problem with lactic acid is that it upsets the body's pH which is the environment for all the cells. Every cell in the body becomes dysfunctional when the pH changes, and if it goes on long enough, the cells will start to die. The more dead cells you have, the more likely you are to have a dead patient. Making ATP anaerobically is a short term compensatory mechanism. You cannot live a long and healthy life anaerobic. You need to find out what is wrong, (is it a problem with ventilation, perfusion, or both?) and fix it before you have a dead patient.

KEEPING THE HEART BEATING

If asked which organ is the most important in the human body, many people will say that the brain is because that is where the essence of the human being resides. The ancient Greeks thought it resided in our liver. I don't know where the human spirit is located, but if you have ever had a brain dead patient, you know that the rest of their body works just fine, thank you. If you have ever had a "heart dead" patient, you know that the rest of the body will only continue to work for minute or two. When I ask what the most important organ in the body is, I'm really asking you which organ kills you first.

When you die, 100% of the time you die from a lethal dysrhythmia. You don't die from hypoxia, you die from the lethal dysrhythmia caused by the hypoxia. You don't die from renal failure, you die from the lethal dysrhythmia caused by the renal failure. When you go, 100% of the time you go from a lethal dysrhythmia. So, let's take a look at what you have to do to keep someone's heart beating.

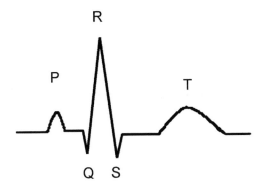

The pQRSt you see running across the EKG screen does not signify squeeze in the heart. It is an *electrical request* for squeeze. It asks *"Please squeeze now if you don't mind."* Most of the time the heart says, *"Sure, I don't mind"* and squeezes, but not always. It is possible to get a beautiful electrical request for squeeze and therefore a beautiful EKG, but still have no squeeze. This is called pulseless electrical activity (PEA). But most of the time when asked, the heart agreeably contracts.

I said it was an *electrical request* for a squeeze, which means you generate electricity in your body. You do that by shifting ions across a semi-permeable membrane. Those are the very same ions you get from fruit, vegetables, and grains. You eat the ions and hope you can retain them long enough to use them.

THE FOUR REQUIREMENTS FOR A HAPPY HEARTBEAT

If you placed an electrode inside a myocardial cell and watched the electricity course through it, this is what you would see on your oscilloscope. This is your action potential.

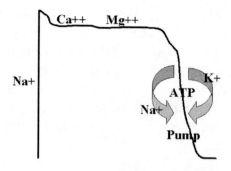

The sharp upstroke is caused by Na+ rushing into the cell, the peak is a Na+ overshoot mediated by K+, the plateau is where Ca++ sustains the squeeze, and Mg++ is used for membrane stability. Now that we have depolarized, we must repolarize, and to do that we need energy. The only energy we have is ATP and we run another Na+ – K+ – ATP pump to shove those ions back against the gradient and get ready for the next heartbeat.

There are four things that must be perfect for the action potential to work and the human heart to beat:

1. You must have a normal pH (the environment for cell function),
2. All the electrolytes must be balanced to generate the action potential,
3. There must be oxygen, and
4. glucose inside the myocardial cell to make ATP to repolarize the cell and get ready for the next beat

One hundred percent of the time when you die, you die from a lethal dysrhythmia caused by an imbalance in one or more of the above requirements for a happy heart beat. Take any disease process you can think of, work your way down to the moment of death, and you will find one or more of the four requirements out of alignment. The end goal of oxygenating and perfusing is that the patient have a normal pH, balanced electrolytes, and oxygen and glucose inside the cell so that that the patient can repolarize his action potential and get ready for the next heartbeat.

DIGITALIS

Earlier, I had said that $Ca++$ sustained the squeeze in the myocardial cell. If you want to increase myocardial contractility, do you suppose that having more $Ca++$ in the cell would do so? Yes, it would, but there is a problem with the $Ca++$. $Ca++$ is linked to $Na+$ and water. To increase myocardial contractility, you want more $Ca++$ to stay behind in the cell, but you don't want the $Na+$ and water to stay. That would cause the cell to swell up and burst. What you need is a drug that poisons the $Na+ - K+ - ATP$ pump on the cell membrane so that the $Na+$ and water is pumped out, but more $Ca++$ is left behind. This drug is called Digitalis. Because of its interaction with the $Na+ - K+ - ATP$ pump, there are 4 things that must be absolutely perfect for a person taking digitalis:

1. There must be a normal pH (the environment for cell function),
2. All the electrolytes must be balanced to generate the action potential,
3. There must be oxygen, and
4. glucose inside the myocardial cell to make ATP to repolarize the cell and get ready for the next beat

If a patient has difficulty with digitalis, it usually signals an electrolyte imbalance, but digitalis does not effect electrolytes. So what happened to the patient's electrolytes?

Back in nursing school when you were trying to answer a test question, there were probably times when you thought to yourself, *"It depends."* You may have gone to the instructor and said, *"The answer to this question depends."* She might have replied, *"You're reading too much into the question."* So you would go back to your seat and make a guess. Well, nothing in nursing/medicine is linear. *"It depends"* is always the right answer.

When considering a situation you must consider all variables—other co-morbid factors, other drugs that may be on board, other insults to the system that may be occurring, the patient's kidneys, his breathing, his nutritional status, and on and on. There are so many things that need to be considered. When trying to determine why a patient is having difficulty with digitalis, consider that it is usually the

27

electrolytes that are off. Though digitalis didn't affect the patient's electrolytes, the Lasix you gave him *with* the digitalis did.

Patients who are CO_2 retaining COPDers, will retain CO_2 and make themselves acidotic. People taking potassium-sparing diuretics can become alkalytic. Based on the four requirements for a happy heart beat and the addition of digitalis, it seems to me that you should never give digitalis to anyone who is a CO_2 retaining COPDer, anyone on potassium-sparing diuretics, anyone who could ever become hypoxic, or anyone who is diabetic. But these are the patients who are most likely to get digitalis! Digitalis is an excellent drug, but it requires a delicate balance in the patient and a vigilant nurse. If you have a patient with an imbalance in any of the four requirements and has digitalis on board, they are at *high* risk for a lethal dysrhythmia and death. You must get it fixed!

Purposes of the Organ Systems | 3

I n school, we studied the functioning of the organ systems, but we seldom looked at the purpose of those organs. What is the purpose of the GI system? It takes food from outside the body, breaks it into little, tiny pieces (those biological substrates) and puts them into the circulatory system. From the circulatory system they go to the cells. Cells use the food you eat to make energy, make other needed substances, and repair your infrastructure. Then you store the remainder on your hips.

What is the purpose of your respiratory system? It brings in air from outside the body, extracts the oxygen, and puts the oxygen into the circulatory system. From the circulatory system it goes to the cells. The cells make ATP out of it. There are chemical reactions in the cells that require oxygen be present for them to occur, but the vast majority of the oxygen you breathe is used to make ATP.

Why will a patient who has stopped breathing die? Because there is no O_2 for ATP to repolarize her action potential. If you can't repolarize your action potential and get ready for the next heart beat to come along, you will have a lethal dysrhythmia and die. The very first ATP that you need to make is that which is required to repolarize the last action potential. Everything else comes after that. So if your patient quits breathing, you must jump in immediately and either get her breathing again or sustain respiration for her before the lethal dys-rhythmia occurs.

What is the purpose of the cardiovascular system? It is a transport media. That is all that it is. It brings the good stuff to the cells and takes the bad stuff away. What is the purpose of the heart? It is the pump that moves the transportation system. If the heart stops beating, good stuff stops coming to the cells, bad stuff stops going away, and very soon you will have dead cells. The more dead cells you get, the more likely you are to get a dead human being.

What is the purpose of the renal system? One purpose is to rid the body of waste. One of those waste products is BUN—blood urea nitrogen. This comes from protein metabolism in the individual cells. When you ask where something comes from in the body, the answer is always from the cells. You can say it comes from the tissues or from the organs, but they are made of cells. Remember, those kidneys are also responsible for balancing your pH, electrolytes, and balancing fluids—three things that can make you real dead real quick.

What is the purpose of the musculo-skeletal system? What advantage is there to being an upright mobile creature as opposed to being a big amoeba lying on the floor? What do we get because we can walk around? Our only energy source in the human body is ATP made of oxygen and glucose. If we are hungry we can go get something to eat. The amoeba has to wait for it to float by. If it doesn't float by, the amoeba starves.

When we go get something to eat, we frequently go get something to drink. We can manipulate and manage our own body's fluid balance. The amoeba survives at the mercy of the fluid around it. If the pond dries up, the amoeba dries up, but we upright mobile creatures can attempt to control our own fluid balance.

We can move to good things, and we can also move away from bad things. If I hear a train coming, I move to get off the train tracks. I will move out of the sun into the pool and order an iced tea from the cute bartender at the in-pool bar before I die of heat stroke. This is a good manipulation of events and environment.

Because I am an upright creature, along with my back ache, I get the ability to see farther and hear better. I can put some of my sensory organs on a stalk and I can rotate them. In this way, I can hear, see, and smell more efficiently than if I was lying on the floor all the time. Being upright creatures gives us advance warning of good and bad things coming our way.

We have fabulous nervous systems—particularly when we are young. In later life it can, at times, leave something to be desired. It is believed that only human beings can predict the future. Can we really predict the future? You bet we can and we don't even need a crystal ball. If you decide to feed your two year old brussels sprouts, do you know what will happen? If your 15 year old daughter calls up and says she is spending the night with her boyfriend, do you know what will happen? If you get on *that* freeway at *that* time of day in *that* city, you know *exactly* what is going to happen.

Because we can predict the future it can save us a lot of grief. Other animals can have a negative experience and learn to avoid the circumstances, but humans can look at a situation and say, "That doesn't look like a good idea to me!" and never have the negative experience. What a wonderful technique for preservation of the species. You don't get on the freeway at 5 pm, and you don't call your mother up and tell her you are spending the night with your boyfriend.

Earlier I had said that you had all kinds of sensors in your body looking at how things were going. What part of your nervous system looks at the input from those sensors and makes adjustments? It is the part of the nervous system that you probably hated studying the most in nursing school. You may have blanked it out of your conscious memory. It is our marvelous, amazing, *autonomic* nervous system.

We have a wonderful system that cranks us up in times of stress and then brings us right back down when the stress is gone. The *sympathetic* and *parasympathetic* nervous systems. Why is it that you need to be cranked back down at all? Why can't you just stay sympathetically stimulated? Because you can't eat enough to generate the energy, repair your infrastructure, and make the stuff to go "full bore" like that. So our system cranks us up in times of stress and brings us right back down when the stress is gone.

Our bodies have changed very little inside since the caveman days. The environment has changed drastically outside, but inside we are pretty much the same as we have always been.

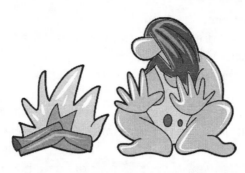

Imagine that you are living in the stone age. It is night time, and you are outside your cave warming your hands at the fire. You have your new cave skins on and you look very sharp tonight. All of a sudden, you hear a twig snap behind you, and you whirl around. Would it be advantageous to increase the blood flow into your brain at this time? Why? What are you going to do with more blood in your brain? Think faster? How does more blood in your brain help you do that? You need oxygen? Oxygen for what? ATP! If you want to fire your neurons faster and heighten your senses, you need more ATP!

To get more oxygen, you breathe faster and deeper, your bronchioles get bigger, and dilating the blood vessels into the brain kicks up the transport system.

So you have your transport mechanism in high gear, and you've thrown in lots of oxygen, but ATP is oxygen plus glucose. So we'd better stop and get a sweet roll. No? Where are you going to get the glucose from? You get the glucose from your stores.

Just what stores are you thinking of? You had better not be thinking of your fat. Your body guards it fat stores carefully. That fat is there for the trek across the Sahara during the famine. Should you be so irresponsible as to loose some of your fat, your body will help you find it again and give you some extra in case you choose to act irresponsibly again. Your fat is your body's last choice when going after energy stores.

The first place you have stores are in the muscle cells themselves. You have three minutes of oxyhemoglobin that will get you up and get you going. In your liver you store glycogen, which can be released into the circulatory system and be used by the cells to make ATP. Where else will you have stores?

It is not unusual for you to go without eating for hours before going to bed, and it is not unusual for you to go without eating for hours after you get up in the morning. What did your body run on all night long while you weren't eating? Your body used the stores contained in the muscle cells themselves. Your body tears down the muscle cells into their little amino acid parts, releases them back into the blood stream, and sends them off to the liver. The liver makes new sugar out of it with a process called *gluconeogenesis*. All night long you run on gluconeogenesis.

The next morning you get up, eat some amino acids for breakfast, and put them right back into your muscle cells. It is a continuous up and down replication process that works beautifully until you make someone NPO. (An abbreviation for the latin term *nil per os*, meaning "nothing by mouth.") If you make someone NPO, his body goes immediately after his muscle cells. Remember that the heart and diaphragm are two large muscles that you don't really want broken down for their stores. This is why nutrition is so important.

Let's get back to our hypothetical cave dweller. The twig snaps and the cave dweller becomes sympathetically stimulated. When you are sympathetically stimulated, do you digest your food? No, this nonessential function slows down. Are sympathetically stimulated people interested in sex? They shouldn't be. They need to be paying attention to their environment!

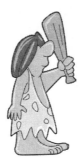

You hear a noise turn around and look, and you see your friend behind you. You can't stay sympathetically stimulated—you need to be *parasympathetically* stimulated. Your heart rate goes down. Your bronchioles get smaller. Do you digest your food? Yes. Are you interested in sex? Perhaps, depending on who it was behind you.

The sympathetic system is "fight or flight," the parasympathetic system is "feed and breed." We were designed to be much more parasympathetically stimulated than sympathetically stimulated. We are frequently too sympathetically stimulated, and we have all kinds of health problems because of it. You were designed for a tropical island, not a hospital.

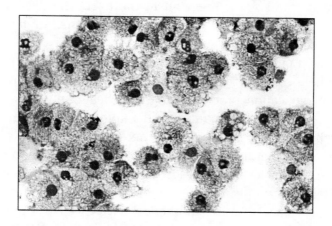

These are macrophages. Did you make them out of the food you eat? Do they use ATP as an energy source? You bet. How well do they work when the body is hypoxic? Not so well. How do they work when the blood sugar is out of adjustment? Not so well. The problem with diabetics and infection is not that they don't have the macrophages—they usually do. The problem is that the macrophages are sluggish because they don't uptake the glucose in the blood the way they should to make ATP and run an active immune system. Diabetics are very prone to infections, especially when they are stressed.

If you want to get your patient back into a state of wellness, two things that you can do to speed them in that direction are to make sure they never become hypoxic (or if they do, get them out of it immediately), and keep tight control of the blood sugar. We are beginning to see patients on the hospital wards with insulin drips going because having a normal blood sugar is key to macrophage functioning and wound healing. Sliding scale coverage is nice, but having a continuous normal blood sugar is even nicer.

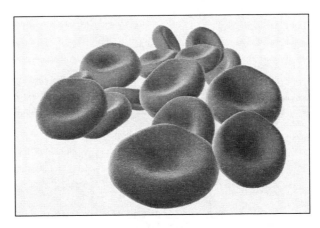

These are red blood cells. Red blood cells are what we use to deliver oxygen to the cells so they can use it to make ATP and so that it can be a catalyst for other chemical reactions. The red blood cells are smooth on the edges so they don't get stuck in places, causing ischemia and infarctions. They also have a dip in the middle that increases the surface area for binding hemoglobin to the oxygen molecules. You could get the same increase in surface area if you bulged the red cell out, but if you bulged them out they would not fit into tight spaces. A red blood cell can literally fold over on itself in a tight space and spring back to normal configuration when the space is larger. They are slick, flexible, and fantastic. This is what we use to deliver oxygen to the cells.

OXYGEN DELIVERY TO THE CELLS

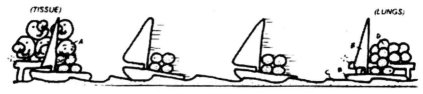

The illustration above goes from the right to the left, not left to right as the words on this page.

The dock represents the lungs, the Os the oxygen molecules, the sail boats are the red blood cells, and the wind in the sails is the blood pressure. If you have functioning lungs, oxygen available, sufficient red blood cells to carry the oxygen, and enough blood pressure to carry it to the target, oxygen is delivered to the tissues. But now, let's get sick. Hypoxia is a symptom of something else going wrong.

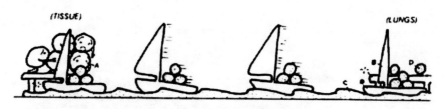

In a hypoxic hypoxia, insufficient oxygen has been delivered to the dock, so insufficient oxygen is loaded onto the red blood cells, and insufficient oxygen is delivered to the tissues. This irritates the heck out of those cells, they go anaerobic, don't work as well, and begin to pump out lactic acid which poisons the environment for all the cells. The treatment for this patient is oxygen. Intubate, tracheostomy, heliOx, *whatever*—you must get oxygen into the patient or he is going to die of a lethal dysrhythmia caused by an inability to repolarize his action potential.

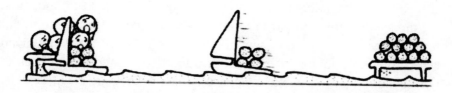

In an anemic hypoxia, there are insufficient red blood cells to carry the oxygen to the cells. The cells couldn't care less why the oxygen didn't arrive, it didn't arrive! The result is the same on the cellular level. The cells get irritated, stop functioning properly, and crank out lactic acid.

What is your treatment? Add some red blood cells to the mixture, right? Maybe, maybe not. I don't think anything has changed more in my nursing career than the decision about who does or who doesn't get a blood transfusion. When I first got out of school, if a patient had a Hematocrit of less than 32 they got a transfusion. Not any more. We had that little problem in the blood supply called the AIDS epidemic and it made us stop and look at the way we gave people blood.

A healthy teenager who suffered a trauma was sent home with an H&H of 15/5. Should this patient have been transfused before he was discharged? Consider that this teenager's bone marrow is in pristine condition. If you want him to make red blood cells, you feed him, and he will make them just as fast as he can. He will be tired and run down for a while, but he won't end up with AIDS, hepatitis, or whatever else we might be passing around in the blood supply. When I got out of school we had hepatitis A, B, and non-A non-B. We are now up to H in the hepatitises. Hepatitis C is not a new disease. It was always there. We didn't know what was causing all that liver failure and liver cancer. We now know it was hepatitis C, and we were passing it around in the blood supply.

Not giving someone a unit of blood is a really swell idea—if you can get away with it. And whether or not you can get away with it depends on three factors.

To Transfuse or Not to Transfuse

1. Who is the patient? What are his reserves? Does he have a lot of co-morbid factors going into the event or was he strong and healthy?

2. What is the nature of the event? Is it over or is it continuing? Was it severe or mild?

3. How much time do you have? If there is time, allow the patient to make his own new blood cells. If there isn't time, transfuse immediately!

A patient in cardiac arrest was admitted to the ER. His hematocrit was 32. For a patient who has just had a cardiac arrest, a hematocrit of 32 is entirely too low. He was promptly given two units of packed red blood cells. A lot of our patients are elderly with poor reserves, and we are more likely to transfuse these patients sooner. It always depends on the patient, the circumstances, and the available time.

If you want to know if a patient is making new red blood cells, take a look at the retic count. A reticulocyte is a brand new red blood cell. If the patient is reticing, you may be less likely to transfuse. We also have erythropoietin these days, which can stimulate someone's hematological stem cells to turn themselves into red blood cells. If a patient is getting EPO or Neupogen, nutrition is crucial. You have to give the patient the biological substrates to make the red cells or they simply can't do it.

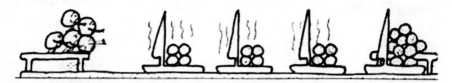

Another form of hypoxia is *stagnant hypoxia* in which there is decreased blood flow, or no wind in the sails. Stagnant hypoxia comes in two forms: total body, called *shock* and localized, called an *infarction*. If you have a patient in shock you must get him out of shock. You need an ACLS book. In the book there is a lovely chapter called *hypotension* with an algorithm that will work you through the problem and get your patient out of shock.

If what you have is a localized infarction, you must reestablish blood flow. You can use balloon angioplasty, clot busters, embolectomies, lasers, roto rooters, *whatever*—you must get blood flowing again or whatever the artery feeds is going to die. No blood flow, no oxygen delivery, no ATP, no sodium potassium pump, and the cell swells up and becomes dysfunctional. If this goes on long enough, the cell lyses and dies. Enough dead cells, you get a dead patient.

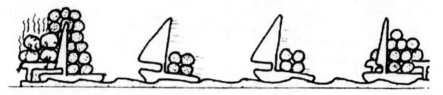

Our last hypoxia is *hystotoxic* hypoxia. In this form of hypoxia, everything is just fine for delivering the oxygen to the cells. The cells themselves are dead from cyanide poisoning and can't utilize the oxygen. For example, patients who receive Nipride (nitroprusside) for extend periods of time can die from cyanide poisoning. It turns out that one of the metabolites of Nipride is cyanide. For this reason we no longer put patients on it for extended periods. We may not always know what we are doing, but we can learn from our mistakes.

Hypoxia is a symptom of a failure to deliver oxygen to the cells where it is used to make ATP. It could be a failure to deliver enough oxygen, a failure of exchange in the lungs, a failure in the transport system, or a failure in the cells ability to uptake the oxygen. Hypoxia is not a diagnosis, it is a symptom of something else—pneumonia, pulmonary embolus, severe anemia, poor blood flow—something that is compromising the delivery of oxygen into the cells. So, if you have a hypoxic patient, as you are treating the hypoxia you ask yourself, "What made this patient hypoxic?" You must find and cure the *cause* of the hypoxia to make the patient anything more than temporarily better.

OXYGEN BINDING CAPACITY

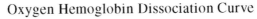

Oxygen Hemoglobin Dissociation Curve

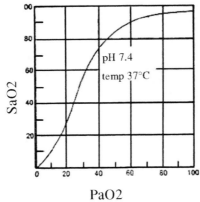

PaO2

Have you ever wondered why it is that oxygen clings to hemoglobin in the lungs, but then lets go when it gets out into the tissues? Even if you've never spent a second thinking about it, there are people who have spent their entire careers thinking about it. It has to do with pH. The environment in the lungs is more alkalytic, and oxygen has an affinity for hemaglobin in an alkalytic environment—it grabs right on. Out in the tissues it is more acidic, and the oxygen lets go—it dissociates. All the oxygen-hemaglobin dissociation curve says is that the amount of oxygen available to the patient's tissues depends on the body's pH.

In the good old days, if we were having a code, the first thing we did after we got some lines into the patient was to slam two amps of bicarb into the patient because he had been acidic. We keep working the code, bagging the patient furiously, and got the first blood gas back showing the patient to be alkalytic. We were very pleased with ourselves because the patient wasn't acidic. Well, turns out being alkalytic is probably worse than being acidic, because less oxygen dissociates from the red blood cells at the tissue level. Your patient needs a normal pH (7.35 to 7.45). So, how much bicarb is given in codes today? None. It is a consideration in a patient with a persistent metabolic acidosis that you cannot ventilate into a normal pH. We may not always know what we are doing, but we are capable of learning on a good day.

SaO2 to PaO2 Conversion Chart

Assuming 37° C and a normal PaCO2

SaO2	PaO2 @ pH 7.3	PaO2 @ pH 7.4	PaO2 @ pH 7.5
97	101	92	84
96	89	82	74
95	82	76	68
94	76	70	61
93	72	66	60
92	68	62	57
91	64	60	54
90	60	58	51
88	59	54	49
86	56	51	47

The above chart is a comparison between O_2 saturation readings and their corresponding arterial blood gas oxygen (PO_2) values. There are three PO_2s—one with a normal pH, one with an acidic pH, and one with an alkalytic pH. Most of us have an O_2 sat of about 97%. If you have a normal pH, that is a PO_2 of 92. A PO_2 of 80 to 100 is normal, so 92 is a good number with a lot of wiggle room. If, however, the pH is alkalytic, it is equivalent to a PO_2 of 84, and if the pH is acidic, it is equivalent to a PO_2 of 101.

See how the pH of the body affects the body's ability to deliver oxygen to the cells? One would think that making the patient acidic would be a good thing if it increases the dissociation of oxygen at the cellular level. It would if that were all you were concerned with, but you must also bind the oxygen to the red blood cell in the first place, and that requires an alkalotic environment in the lungs. Your patient needs a normal pH for the system to work correctly. However, in a time of slow blood flow and shock, oxygen is released quicker from the hemoglobin molecule. Another one of those nice compensatory mechanisms trying to keep you alive.

We frequently begin putting oxygen on patients with a O_2 sat of 92. That corresponds to a PO_2 of 62—if there is a normal pH. It's even worse if there isn't. 80 to 100 is a normal PO_2. Why would you let someone get this low before putting oxygen on him? Is there any group of patients for whom this could be a good number? Sure. For elderly people dying of heart and lung disease, this could be the best they have been in six weeks. When you look at numbers, there is no such thing as a right or "normal" number. It always depends on who the patient is. For someone with end-stage lung disease, an O_2 sat of 92 could be wonderful.

After a while, we begin to think that normals for the types of patients we take care of the most are normals for everyone. They are not. They are only normal for that particular kind of patient.

One of the most frequent patients in a hospital today are elderly people dying of heart and lung disease. A few months of taking care of these patients and you begin to think that their normals are normal for the entire patient population. Be careful. Don't extrapolate normals from this group to any other group. They don't fit.

A high school football player was admitted to the hospital with a ruptured appendix. He had peritonitis, so the nurses recognized that atelectasis would be a real problem for this patient. To counter this, the nurses got out an incentive spyrometer and earnestly went to work on this patient's lungs. He was pulling a liter and a half on the spyrometer! The nurses were used to patients pulling 700 cc, 850 cc. They were amazed and gratified at their patient's progress until day three post op when the morning's chest x-ray showed massive atelectasis! "But why?" they asked. The high school football player should have been pulling 2 and a half liters! The one and a half liters was sub-maximal effort, but to the nurses used to sick old people with bad hearts and bad lungs, it looked wonderful. Always consider the patient. Who is this person? What are their "normals"? What are their reserves?

Numerous changes happen in your body as you get older. If you are over 30 years old (and if you aren't this is what you will get for your thirtieth birthday) speed of conduction in the AV node of your heart will start to slow down, so that by the time you are a little old lady or little old man you could have a first-degree AV block show up on your EKG and it could possibly be normal for you. Contractility of your heart and oxygen-binding capacity will begin to decrease yearly (which is why your exercise capacity has dropped off) so that by the time you are a little old lady of little old man—*and are sedentary*—you could have a low oxygen saturation and it could be normal for you.

Being sedentary is a crucial component. If your patient was an 80-year-old marathon runner, would you expect to see a low sat? Of course not. If the patient walked the dog for a mile a day or was out puttering in the garden or garage, would you expect to see a low sat? No. You have to be sedentary to have a low sat (assuming nothing else is causing it). In our hospitals and care facilities we see mostly elderly, sedentary people in the last years of their lives dying of heart and lung disease. Their normals are not normals for the general population. If I am in your hospital with a sat of 92%, please come see why I am not breathing. I should never have a sat of 92% unless I am in trouble.

Throughout our schooling we have learned that anything greater than 90 is a good thing. So if we see 92, we may think it is the bottom end of normal. In fact, it may be a severe hypoxia. A normal PO_2 is 80 to 100, but that PO_2 of 80 corresponds to an O_2 sat of 95%. The sat of 92% *might* be OK, but consider who it is that you are letting go that low. Remember that every big and little thing in the body requires ATP as an energy source and that it is made of glucose and *oxygen*. A hypoxic patient means a dysfunctional *everything*—including the cardiac action potential.

Blood
Gasses

4

Acid (CO_2) + Base (HCO_3) = pH

<u>Normals</u>

pH	7.35 – 7.45
PCO_2	35 – 45
Bicarb	22 – 26
PO_2	80 – 100

There are two things of primary importance regarding blood gasses: acid base balance and oxygenation. There are more things to be seen on the ABG, but we are going to consider the two most important. The acid base balance is the balance between the acid and the base in our bodies. The principal acid is CO_2 and the main base is our bicarbonate. The balance between the two gives the body its pH, which should be 7.35 to 7.45. If the number is larger than 7.4, it is called an alkalosis, if the number is less than 7.35 it is an acidosis.

The PCO_2 is the acid load, and the value should be 35 to 45. If there is an imbalance in the CO_2, we say there is a respiratory problem.

The bicarbonate should be 22 to 26. If there is an imbalance in the bicarbonate, we say the patient has a metabolic problem. Oxygenation is represented by the PO_2 which should be 80 to 100.

This is a good time to talk about oxygenation and O_2 saturation. Oxygen delivery to the cells depends on much more than saturation of the red blood cells. If you have two red blood cells and both are maximally oxygenated, the O_2 sat will read 100%. It is nice that both are carrying as much oxygen as possible, but it is no where near enough to meet the metabolic needs of the body. Delivering oxygen to the body's cells depends on the number of red blood cells, their quality, availability of oxygen, pH of the body, hormones, metabolic conditions, and blood flow. Percent of oxygen saturation is just one piece of the puzzle, not the whole picture.

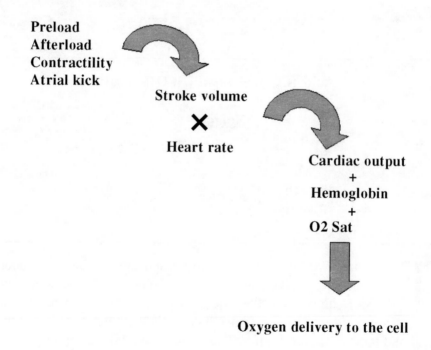

Preload
Afterload
Contractility
Atrial kick

Stroke volume

✗

Heart rate

Cardiac output
+
Hemoglobin
+
O2 Sat

Oxygen delivery to the cell

In the following blood gasses we are going to evaluate numbers, but also ask ourselves what could be causing the situation and what we need to do to rectify it.

NORMAL CHEST X-RAY

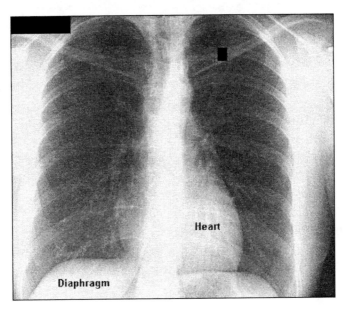

Heart

Diaphragm

BLOOD GAS EXAMPLES

ABG #1		
pH	7.52
PCO2	35.0
Bicarb	28.0
PO2	117

The pH of 7.52 is greater than 7.45, giving the patient an alkalosis. The CO_2 of 35.0 is the lower end of normal, but the bicarbonate of 28 is high, so our patient has a metabolic problem. It is a metabolic alkalosis, because the pH is greater that 7.45 and the imbalance occurs in the bicarbonate not the PCO_2.

The patient's PO_2 is 117. We would like to know if this patient is on oxygen or not. I have wondered for years how high a person could run his PO_2 by hyperventilating on room air. The answer is about 110, although I have heard of a young DKA patient who hyperventilated himself into the 120s on room air. There is always someone who can do it better than anyone else.

This patient has a PO_2 of 117. Is he on oxygen? Most likely. OK, how much oxygen? You can't make any judgments about his ability to oxygenate himself until you know how much he is on. Maybe he has 2 liters of oxygen going giving him a PO_2 of 117. That is one piece of information. What if he has 100% oxygen going, giving you a PO_2 of 117? That is another piece of information.

How much should a patient's PO_2 change when the FiO_2 is changed? The PO_2 should be about 3–4 times what the FiO_2 is. For example if you put a patient on 100% oxygen, you should see a PO_2 of between 300 and 400. If you don't, you have a hypoxic patient, because he is not oxygenating as well as expected. *"But,"* you say, *"a PO_2 of 80 to 100 is normal and 117 is above normal. How can the patient be hypoxic?"* It is a matter of what you have versus what is expected. If the ratio of FiO_2 to PO_2 is off, something is happening. This is another early sign of impending doom. Patients shouldn't need oxygen to have a normal PO_2. *"It's only 2 liters,"* you say. But it shouldn't be anything. Our lungs have tremendous reserve capability. If you need any oxygen at all to have a "normal" PO_2, you have a problem.

Let's look at the concept of *Normal Values.* Normals apply to well, healthy individuals breathing room air with a normal respiratory rate, under normal conditions. As we work the rest of the ABGs, we will begin to question the viability of normals. Remember, everything always depends.

X-RAY #1

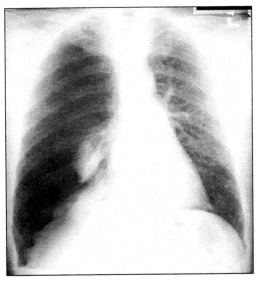

What is wrong in this chest x ray? Answer after the next ABG.

ABG #2		
pH	7.18
PCO$_2$	56.0
Bicarb	22.0
PO$_2$	41.0

In this gas we have a pH of 7.18 which is acidic, a PCO$_2$ of 56 which is high, and a bicarbonate that is the bottom end of normal. An acidic pH and an abnormal PCO$_2$ gives us a respiratory acidosis. One of the things you can tell from a blood gas is how long the event has been going on. You cannot walk around with an abnormal pH. This pH is out of sync because of the large acid (CO$_2$) load. To compensate for this, the body will retain a lot of its base (bicarbonate) and swing the pH back to normal. The body retains the bicarbonate in the kidneys, and this can take days. Is this an acute or chronic situation? Has the body had days to retain bicarbonate, compensate for the huge acid load and return the pH to normal? No. So this is an acute respiratory acidosis and not something that has been going on for some time.

47

The PO₂ is 41. What is this patient not doing? He's not breathing, and I sincerely hope you noticed it before the gas came back. You have a patient who is acutely *not* breathing and he needs your help. Some stimulation, a few drugs, an ET tube—*something,* or he is going to be dead.

Speaking of dead, how do you get that way? From a lethal dysrhythmia. The causes of this patient's lethal dysrhythmia are both the pH and hypoxia. This patient is screaming toward a lethal dysrhythmia just as fast as he can via two separate pathways, and if you don't oxygenate and perfuse at the same time to keep his pH normal, his electrolytes balanced, and O₂ and glucose inside the cell being used to make ATP, he will be successful.

ANSWER X-RAY #1: In the patient's left lung (remember it is a mirror image) there are little white lines called lung markings. They represent the pulmonary vasculature. You can see them all the way up and down the lung. Look at the right lung. Do you see any lung markings in the base of the lung? Up between the ribs? Over by the heart is the patient's collapsed lung. This is a pneumothorax.

X-Ray #2

What about this chest x-ray? The answer follows the next ABG.

ABG #3		
pH	7.37
PCO_2	55.0
Bicarb	31.0
PO_2	65

In this gas we have a normal pH, a high PCO_2, and a high bicarbonate. This a respiratory acidosis as seen by the high CO_2, but the pH is normal because this patient has had days to retain bicarbonate in his kidneys and swing his pH back to normal. This is, therefore, a patient that is used to having his PCO_2 high—a CO_2 retaining COPDer. He retains bicarbonate and swings his pH back to normal, because you must have a normal pH for the cells to function properly, and life is about appropriately functioning cells.

This patient is a CO_2 retaining COPDer. We need to differentiate the retainer from the average COPDer. In the great category of COPD there is a small subcategory called retainers. They are few in number when compared to the whole because CO_2 exchanges across the membrane 20 times faster than O_2. By the time patients are retaining CO_2, they have destroyed so much of their lung tissue that they will, 1) never have a normal PO_2, and 2) not live very long. They do however, flood into our hospitals during the last few years of their lives, making it seem that all COPDers are also retainers. This is not true, but it can seem so if you look at our patient populations.

In this ABG the patient has a PO_2 of 65. A PO_2 of 80 to 100 is normal. Shall we turn up the FiO_2? Is our patient a CO_2 retaining COPDer? Yes, you can see it with the high CO_2 and the normal pH. This means the condition had been present for the days required to retain bicarb in the kidneys and swing the pH back to normal.

What causes a CO_2 retaining COPDer's only drive to breathe? You and I have two drives to breathe. One, if our PCO_2 goes up we breathe faster, and two, if our PO_2 goes down we breathe faster. If you have a chronically high PCO_2 you blunt the CO_2 receptors, and they don't respond any more. Now your only drive to breathe is hypoxia. You need to make sure the CO_2 retaining COPDer stays hypoxic. The question is, how hypoxic do they need to be? You don't want your patient to be any more hypoxic than he absolutely has to be, because ATP runs everything in the body and ATP requires oxygen. Nothing is functioning properly in the body of a hypoxic patient.

The mistake we make with ABGs for CO_2 retainers is that we look at the PO_2 of 65 and say, "Oh, he's a retainer. He needs to be hypoxic so leave him alone." Always take the ABG results to the bedside and see how the patient is doing with those numbers. If he is playing cards with his wife, is this a good number for him? If he is confused, weak, and hostile is this a good PO_2 for him? It always depends on how the patient is doing with the numbers that determines if the gas is good for him. Maybe he wants his PO_2 a little closer to 70—never normal—but maybe he could use half, one, or maybe 2 liters FiO_2 for optimal functioning. Don't make these patients struggle to breathe any more than they absolutely have to. Life is already hard enough.

ANSWER X-RAY #2: This heart is entirely too large. The width of the heart should be approximately half the width of the chest cavity. This is cardiomeglia.

X-RAY #3

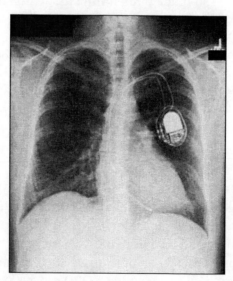

What do you see in this x-ray? Answer follows the next ABG.

ABG #4		
pH		7.53
PCO$_2$		26.0
Bicarb		22.0
PO$_2$		162

This gas shows a patient with an alkalytic pH, a low PCO$_2$, and a normal bicarbonate. This represents a respiratory alkalosis because the PCO$_2$ is low and therefore responsible for the high pH. Respiratory alkalosis frequently causes hyperventilating in a patient. The most common cause of hyperventilating is *not* anxiety, it is hypoxia. But hypoxia will make a patient very anxious. Sometimes we give patients a psychological diagnosis without ruling out hypoxia as a cause of their behavior. However, a PO$_2$ of 162 does not indicate hypoxia, so that cannot be a cause of this patient's hyperventilation.

You may also see values like this with an acute cardiac event. In this event, you have a patient whose heart isn't pumping as well as it should and therefore isn't delivering oxygen to the tissues in adequate amounts. The tissues become hypoxic and they will send a chemical message to the pneumotaxic center in the brain requesting the patient to breathe faster. Because the lungs are normal, the increase in respiration causes the patient to blow off CO$_2$ with the resultant respiratory alkalosis.

Our patient has a PO$_2$ of 162. Our normal PO$_2$ is 80 to 100. Should we turn the FiO$_2$ down? Make no judgments about what to do with a gas until you know the circumstances. Is this patient in the midst of a cardiac event? If he is, are you going to turn his oxygen down? Of course not; you would likely precipitate his lethal dysrhythmia and death. Circumstances are crucial in the decision making process. Remember, normals are normal for well, healthy people under normal circumstances, not for people in the throes of a cardiac crisis. You give the patient all the oxygen he needs to help him through the event, *then* you turn the oxygen down.

ANSWER X-RAY #3: This patient has a pacemaker showing a single lead in the heart. Note the bipolar electrodes in the atrium and the single electrode in the ventricle. Look for the tip of it in the right ventricle. This pacemaker system senses atrial depolarizations and can pace or sense in the ventricle. We call this an A-V sequential pacemaker.

X-Ray #4

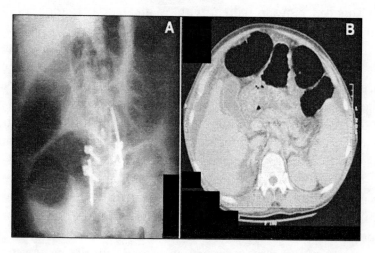

This is an abdominal x-ray and CT scan of the same patient. How do things look to you? Answer follows the ABG.

ABG #5		
pH	7.10
PCO$_2$	35.0
Bicarb	11.0
PO$_2$	338

    The acidic pH in this gas is being caused by a very low bicarbonate and is therefore called a metabolic acidosis. Is it acute or chronic? If the pH still out of whack, then it is acute. Things that can cause a metabolic acidosis include diabetic keto acidosis and ion gap acidosis from an electrolyte imbalance. But, by far, the largest number of metabolic acidosis are caused by lactic acidosis because of a failure to oxygenate, a failure to perfuse, or a failure to oxygenate and perfuse at the same time.

Our patient has a PO₂ of 338. Can we all agree to turn his FiO₂ down? Is he well and healthy, or is he in crisis? We know he is in crisis from looking at the pH. The most likely thing to have caused the pH to be so low is a lactic acidosis from a failure to oxygenate, a failure to perfuse, or a failure to oxygenate and perfuse. We see his oxygenation is good with the PO₂ of 338. It is failure to perfuse, shock, that is the most likely cause of his low pH. If this patient has a low blood pressure you aren't going to turn his FiO₂ down; you would precipitate his lethal dysrhythmia. Always ask yourself what the circumstances are surrounding the values. We are going to make this patient better, get him out of crisis, stabilize him, and *then* turn his FiO₂ down.

ANSWER X-RAY #4: In the flat plate of the abdomen, hardware is visible in the patient's spine. We also can see large dilated loops of bowel. The CT is a sagittal view through the body and the gas trapped in this patient's colon is clearly evident. This is a patient with toxic megacolon.

X-RAY #5

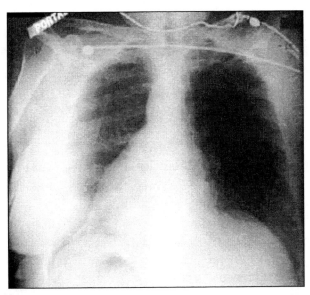

What do you see here? Answer follows the blood gas.

ABG #6		
pH		7.46
PCO$_2$		32.0
Bicarb		22.0
PO$_2$		69.0

In this gas, the pH is slightly alkalytic, but barely so. We can see that the cause for the pH is the low PCO$_2$, resulting in a rather mild respiratory alkalosis. It is an acute situation because the bicarbonate is normal and the pH is abnormal. The patient is suddenly breathing more rapidly. Remember, the most common cause of hyperventilation is hypoxia. Is this patient hypoxic? Yes, the PO$_2$ is 69 and 80 to 100 is normal. In a previous example I said that the PO$_2$ of 65 might be a good number for that patient. We know that this PO$_2$ of 69 is abnormal for this patient because he is hyperventilating. We have a patient with an acute hypoxic event.

But the gas is rather unremarkable, isn't it? No, not at all. This gas screams acute hypoxic event in a fairly well, healthy person with good compensatory mechanisms. The younger and healthier a person is, the more able they are to hyperventilate themselves into a fairly normal gas in the face of a sudden hypoxia.

A student nurse goes into the ER complaining of shortness of breath, chest discomfort, and sudden anxiety while studying for the next day's test. They shoot a CXR that shows clear lungs, and they draw a gas which comes back with a pH 7.48, PCO$_2$ 31, bicarbonate 22, and PO$_2$ 82. The ER staff informs the student that she is having an anxiety attack and sends her back to the dorm to rest and calm down.

The student feels something is really wrong inside and she calls her mother seeking advice. The mother calls the family physician who instructs the mother to tell the daughter to go back to the ER immediately and tell the physician that her family has a hyper coagulable syndrome, causing them to make clots at the drop of a hat. Upon further workup it is found that the student has thrown a pulmonary embolus so large that it occludes one entire lung. Because she was so young and so healthy she was able to hyperventilate herself into an almost normal gas in the face of a catastrophic event.

The younger and healthier you are the more likely you are to be able to hyperventilate yourself into a fairly normal gas. The older and sicker you are the quicker you crash. Remember, the number one cause of hyperventilation is hypoxia and that hypoxia makes you very anxious. You shouldn't have to hyperventilate to give yourself a normal PO_2.

ANSWER X-RAY #5 How does the position of the heart in the chest appear to you? The apex of the ventricles is pointed the wrong way. *Laevocardia* is the normal cardiac position with the heart in the left side of the chest, *dextrocardia* implies the heart is predominantly in the right hemi-thorax, and in mesocardia the heart lies in the midline. This x-ray is of dextrocardia.

X-Ray #6

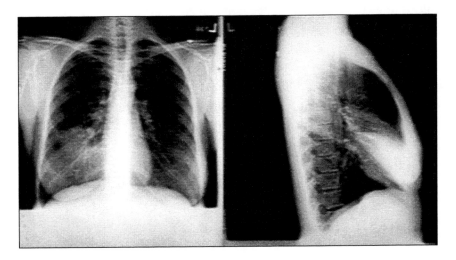

PA and Lateral films of the same patient. What do you see? Answer follows the next ABG.

ABG #7		
pH		7.06
PCO₂		40.3
Bicarb		1.4
PO₂		86.0

This patient has a *very* acidic pH caused by the *very* low bicarbonate. It has happened quickly and his respiratory rate isn't able to respond and bring the pH back to normal. We have an acute metabolic acidosis. The PO₂ is 86; 80 to 100 is normal. Do you want to change the FiO₂? Turn it up maybe? Is this patient in crisis? Yes. How do you know? Look at the pH. This patient is getting ready to have his lethal dysrhythmia caused by the severe acidosis. Abnormal pH is one of the four things that can lead to a lethal dysrhythmia and this is a *very* abnormal pH. The most common cause of a metabolic acidosis is lactic acidosis caused by a failure to oxygenate, a failure to perfuse, or a failure to oxygenate and perfuse at the same time.

Does this gas belong to a well, healthy individual? Do normals apply in this acute crisis? The most likely thing causing this acidosis is a low blood pressure. If this patient is in shock, do you want him to be left with a *normal* PO₂? No. You want to shove it just as high as you can get it, make the patient all better, then turn it down after you have corrected the problem and stabilized the patient.

ANSWER X-RAY #6: PA view of a patient with right middle lobe pneumonia, showing consolidation and loss of the right heart silhouette. The lateral view clearly shows the wedge shaped middle lobe and not the lower lobe is involved. This is why chest films are ordered PA and Lateral whenever possible.

X-Ray #7

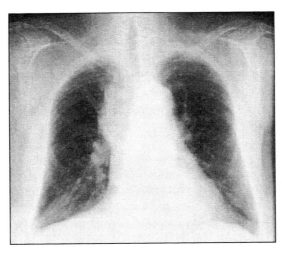

This patient presented with a persistent productive cough of 3 months duration. What do you see?

ABG #8		
pH		**7.35**
PCO₂		**60.0**
Bicarb		**34.0**
PO₂		**101.0**

In this gas, two abnormals make a normal. There is a high PCO_2 representing a large acid load and a high bicarbonate representing a large base load. The two of them compensate for each other and result in a normal pH. This is another gas belonging to a CO_2 retaining COPDer. The PCO_2 is high at 60 and the chronic component is seen in the time required for the kidney to retain bicarbonate and swing the pH back to normal. This patient is used to having his CO_2 up and has nicely balanced himself.

He has a PO_2 of 101. Normal is 80 to 100. Do you want to change his FiO_2? Does it depend on how he is doing with these numbers? He's doing great. He's watching *Millionaire Survivor Apprentice Bachelor* on TV, and he is laughing and having a good time. Do you want to turn his oxygen down? Yes, absolutely.

Is this patient a CO_2 retaining COPDer? Absolutely. That means that his only drive to breathe is hypoxia, and he is not hypoxic with a PO_2 of 101.

I said he was doing fine, and he is right now, but CO_2 narcosis usually takes hours. Hypoxia kills in seconds to minutes. Some retainers will crash and burn quickly, but most spend hours going into CO_2 narcosis.

A CO_2 retaining COPDer in the last year of her life came into the hospital to be intubated, cleaned out, and set right about once a month. On this particular day, she called 911, but when the paramedics got there they didn't need to intubate her. She was in crisis, so they gave her 100% oxygen, which was exactly the right thing to do. They transported her to the ER where she got further treatment, but did not need intubation. The 100% oxygen was still flowing.

The ER decided after treatment that not only did they not need to intubate her, she did not require the ICU either, so they called for a room on the floor. The high flow oxygen was still going. Hours later, she arrived on the floor with her high flow oxygen still going. She was admitted, the nurse brought her lunch, she ate, turned over, and went to sleep. She awakened several hours later in the ICU on a ventilator with a PCO_2 of 120. *You cannot leave the high flow oxygen on.*

ANSWER X-RAY #7: PA view of a patient with a large cell carcinoma of the upper lobe of the right lung, presenting as a very large right upper lobe mass.

X-Ray #8

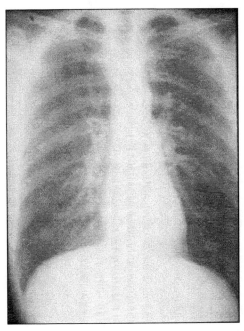

Sometimes x-ray reports come back saying the patient has hyper-inflated lungs. These lungs come way down beyond what would be expected. The heart normally sits towards the left side of the chest, but if the lungs hyperinflate, it becomes more midline, and the diaphragm drops way down.

How much oxygen should you give a CO_2 retaining COPDer?

In the good old days after we discovered that there was such a thing as a CO_2 retaining COPDer, we were taught that if you gave them too much oxygen they went to sleep and didn't wake up. So the word went out that all COPDers could have 2 liters of oxygen and *no more than* 2 liters of oxygen. The educational campaign was massive and complete. Everyone heard that COPDers were to be limited to an FiO_2 of 2 liters and no more and we all complied.

Then someone came along and did a study and found that if you limit these patients to 2 liters of oxygen at the time of the exerbation of their COPD, they died in large numbers from lethal dysrhythmias because they could not repolarize their action potentials. So then the word went out that COPDers could have all the oxygen they needed when they were in crisis. Unfortunately, the group that put out the 2 liter rule had a much better educational campaign that the group trying to take it back. What we are left with is a great deal of confusion in some circles about how much oxygen you should give a COPDer.

Remember, that the only patients who have trouble with oxygen are CO_2 *retaining* COPDers. The average COPDer has no trouble with oxygen. Remember also that we are talking about the short run—the patient in crisis. On top of his COPD, this patient also has fluid overload, pneumonia, an asthma attack, or something else that is exerbating his lung disease. His life is in danger from a lethal dysrhythmia caused by an abnormal pH, an imbalance in his electrolytes, or not having oxygen and glucose in the cells being used to make ATP.

Let's say I am a CO_2 retaining COPDer. On a good day I have a PO_2 of 75. It will never be normal, I am a retainer and my disease has destroyed a great deal of my lung tissue. I have now had an exerbation of my COPD and my PO_2 drops to 60. Do I have a drive to breathe? Am I hypoxic? You bet I am. I am *severely* hypoxic. Since you understand about ATP formation and the action potential, you give me 100% oxygen because you don't want me to die from a lethal dysrhythmia, and I thank you. I'm not ready to go just yet.

We keep working on me and the next gas comes back with a PO_2 of 65. Do I have a drive to breathe? Am I hypoxic? Yes, I am. We keep working and the next gas has a PO_2 of 68. Do I have a drive to breathe? Sure, I'm still hypoxic for me. For the next gas, the PO_2 is 72. Do I have a drive to breathe? Yes. On the next gas, the PO_2 is 76. Do I have a drive to breathe? No, I have exceed my normal of 75. Actually, you needed to start paying attention to me when the PO_2 was 72. But from 60 all the way to 72 I needed 100% oxygen to keep from dying from a lethal dysrhythmia. From 72 to 75 the 2 liter rule applies, and when you reach my normal, it is whatever I am on normally, whether that be room air, half a liter, 2 liters, or whatever. But if you limit me to 2 liters of oxygen at the time of the exerbation of my COPD when I am so horribly hypoxic, I will most likely not make it through the event.

Hypoxia	Normal for Patient	CO$_2$ narcosis
confused, restless, agitated, combative		somnolent

When you observe behavior of patients you can get some clues as to the status of their oxygenation. People who are hypoxic are confused, restless, agitated, and combative. Please—*never* sedate anyone for being confused, restless, agitated or combative until you can prove that this particular episode of confused, restless, agitated and combative is not being driven by hypoxia.

If you had a patient who is a raving lunatic or who sundowns at 7 pm every night, and at 7:01 pm these patients are confused, restless, agitated, and combative, the patient have thrown a pulmonary embolus, developed pneumonia, or be having an MI. So *always* make sure the patient's behavior isn't being driven by hypoxia *before* you sedate him. Sedating hypoxic patients can kill them.

CO$_2$ narcosis produces a somnolent patient, which is a 180-degree difference from the hypoxic patient. One would think that you could never confuse the two, but patients continue to come into the hospital having not seen the above representation and therefore don't know how to fall into neat categories. Sometimes you just don't know. "Should I or should I not give O$_2$?" When in doubt, always use oxygen until data tells you otherwise. Hypoxia kills in seconds to minutes; CO$_2$ narcosis usually takes hours. The beauty of oxygen is that you can always take it off, but you may not get the patient back from a hypoxic code.

The Heart

5

I n your heart there are a series of valves. The purpose of the valves is to direct the blood flow. When the heart squeezes, it use ATP as an energy source, of which there is a finite—not infinite—amount. When the heart squeezes, you want the blood to move out in the proper direction, not back in the direction that it came from. To do so would waste energy. To direct the blood flow in the direction that you want it to go, the heart is equipped with a series of valves. The mitral and tricuspid valve are just little tissue paper things with little structural form. The leaflets are attached via chordae tendineae (like parachute harnesses) to a structure called a papillary muscle that rises up out of the myocardium. When the heart squeezes, the blood is sent backward with the same force it is pushed forward. But the papillary muscle *also* contracts and pulls the valve leaflets down nice and tight, and that ensures the blood is forced out the right way.

These papillary muscles are made of cells, and cells have with sodium-potassium pumps that need to be run, infrastructure that needs to be repaired, and ATP that needs to be generated. The requirements for all of this are brought into the papillary muscle cells by perfusion in the myocardium. If you have an area of the heart that is ischemic, it will not squeeze as well as the rest of the heart. If that ischemia includes a papillary muscle, it will not pull down as tightly as the other papillary muscles. In your stethoscope that sounds like a murmur.

A new onset murmur should be considered a medical emergency until proven otherwise. If a papillary muscle is ischemic, it becomes dysfunctional, but if the ischemia goes on long enough or is severe enough, the patient can rupture that papillary muscle. Now you have a valve leaflet blowing in the breeze. This occurs most often on the left side of the heart where the pressures are higher, and it frequently affects the mitral valve. When this happens, only half the blood goes out the aorta when the heart squeezes. (There goes half your cardiac output.) The other half goes directly back into the patient's lungs giving him an acute 4+ pulmonary edema. This is a catastrophe your patient probably will not survive. The way you fix this problem is with a mitral valve replacement or repair, but first you have to get the patient stable enough to get to the operating room for the surgery.

Time is of the essence. Once the papillary muscle is ruptured the horse is out of the barn. The problem needs to be detected *before* the rupture. You hear the problem coming with a new onset murmur. If you put your stethoscope on a patient's chest and you hear a murmur that no one ever heard before, your first thought may be, *"I made a mistake. There's nothing there."* Instead, if you hear a murmur that no one has ever hear before, get other people in the room to listen. If it *is* a new onset murmur, it can herald papillary muscle rupture.

Cardiac patients are the kind of patients most likely to rupture a papillary muscle, particularly those having inferior events. But did you know that as many as 30% of people having MIs never have a symptom that we recognize as an MI? This is called *silent* ischemia. It is so prevalent that there is even a *Journal of Silent Ischemia.* A man goes in for his yearly physical, and after the EKG, the doctor asks him when he had his MI. The patient doesn't remember an MI, but he did have a bad case of the flu last June. That *was* the MI. So the patient admitted with pneumonia or a small bowel obstruction can also have an undetected MI and papillary muscle rupture. If you do indeed have a new onset murmur, you need a doctor right now.

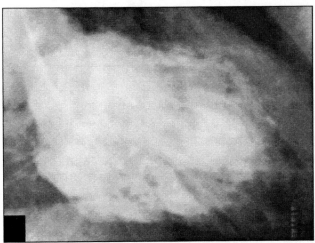

Diastole as seen on an LV gram

Have you ever wondered how the blood pumped from the left heart manages to make it over to the right heart? *"Well,"* you say, *"You push it from the left heart with a high pressure and it ends up in the right heart with a low pressure."* Yes, but that's not the main driving force. You do indeed push it from the left heart with a high pressure, but you push it out into the aorta. The aorta is a large vessel, but the vessels get progressively smaller until they are capillaries only one cell thick. Then the vessels get progressively larger before emptying the blood into the right heart. You can't push all the way through that kind of plumbing.

If you have an intact column of fluid, which is what our cardio-vascular system is, it isn't so much that you push with the high pressure as it is that you draw with the low pressure. Maintaining the low pressure in the right heart is crucial to getting the blood to return. The heart sits in the chest, which is a low pressure system. When we take in a breath, we drop the pressures in the chest and aid the return of blood into the right heart. If anything were to increase the pressures in the chest, it could keep the blood from returning to the heart—things like sucking chest wounds, tension pneumothoraxes, PEEP on a venti-lator, or pulmonary hypertension. These things can overcome the abil-ity of the blood to return to the right heart.

Imagine a motorcyclist out for a ride on a beautiful spring day. He hits a pot hole and is flying through the air at 20 miles per hour when he sees an approaching stop sign and decides to reach out and grab it. Bad idea. He is now lying on the ground and his blood supply is lying on the ground next to him. He does not have an intact column of fluid. In order to save his life, you must plug the hole and fill him back up to give him an intact column of fluid.

The next thing our motorcyclist has to have is a distensible heart. When you pour blood into the heart it has to get bigger. If it doesn't, we have a serious problem, because you cannot get out more than you were able to get in. The heart may be prevented from distending by things like restrictive cardiomyopathy, restrictive pericarditis, or pressures in the wrong place, as in cardiac tamponade.

An example of restrictive cardiomyopathy is amyloidosis. Once I had a patient whose chest x-ray looked like he had gravel all around his heart. He had a chronic pericardial inflammation that he put calcium into. Calcium does not distend, so he had a restrictive pericarditis.

In cardiac tamponade there is so much fluid in the sac surrounding the heart that it pushes up on the walls of the ventricles, and they can't distend. There's often nothing wrong with the heart itself. If you put a needle into the pericardial sac and withdraw the fluid, the heart works just fine. It is a matter of pressures in the right places.

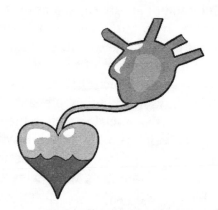

If you have an intact column of fluid, a distensible heart, and pressures in the right place, you get the first part of diastole: passive filling. The second part of diastole is an active filling. The atria are going to contract, and when they do, they are capable of pushing as much as 40% more volume down into the ventricle. This is called the atrial kick. This reserve is a part of the sympathetic response—fight or flight. As you are sitting quietly, your atrial kick is giving you little of your total cardiac output—10 to 15%—because you don't need it. But if you should have to jump up and run, it can give you as much as 40% more cardiac output.

What a tremendous reserve. It has been said that a patient in the unit, post-op, septic, on a vent requires the same amount of energy as a person continually running four-minute miles. If you were running four-minute miles, would you want your atrial kick? Of course you would. Dysrhythmias that can take away the atrial kick include a-fib, a-flutter, junctional, ventricular, and some of the blocks. Any time you don't have one 'p' in front of every QRS you have lost the atrial kick and potentially 40% of the total cardiac output.

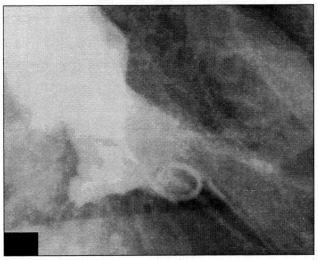

Systole as seen on an LV gram

We've had passive filling and gotten our atrial kick. It is now time for systole. A student once asked me, *"Can you die with a pacemaker in?"* Of course you can. At this point I realized that I had told the students all about ATP, those four conditions, and the action potential, but what I had forgotten to tell them was that if the four conditions of normal pH, balanced electrolytes, oxygen and glucose inside the cell being used to make ATP are not met in the individual myocardial cell, it will not respond to the electrical request for squeeze. The good stuff comes to the myocardial cells because of coronary circulation. It brings the good stuff in and takes the bad stuff away. If you want good, brisk systole, you must have good, brisk coronary circulation. This is why we spend so much time revascularizing patient's hearts.

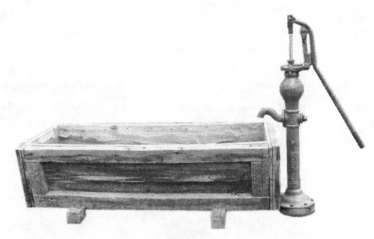

Let's say that you and your horse, Trigger, live out in the desert wasteland. Trigger has osmoreceptors and an active thirst mechanism and he will need to drink water. To supply the water you have a horse trough which you fill with an old fashion hand crank pump. These pumps differ from faucets. When you turn a faucet on, the water runs until you turn the faucet off, but with a hand pump, the water only comes out when you push down on the handle. With every stroke downward on the handle, a certain volume of water comes out, and nothing happens until you push down again. We will call the volume that comes out the *stroke volume* and how fast you push the *rate*.

Everything is just fine for you and Trigger, until one day you notice that when you push down on the handle, less volume comes out. Trigger considers this to be your personal problem—he wants his horse trough full. Now you are going to need to push faster to get the same total volume out.

To detect the source of the problem, you get out your fiber optic scope and snake it down into the well and see that the well is running dry. This requires moving on to Plan B. Plan B is to drill yourself another well directly into your neighbor's aquifer which is brimming over with water. She hates you and is pretty sure this is exactly what you have done. Now every time you push down on the handle, water gushes out all over the place. If she can see extra water all over the ground, she will know that you are into her well. Now to keep the horse trough full but not overflowing, you have to turn the rate down. Or, get another horse. Or, give Lasix to Trigger and he will deposit the extra water all over the ranch.

Cardiac Output = Heart Rate × Stroke Volume

Cardiac output equals heart rate times stroke volume, and if anything affects stroke volume, you see a compensatory rise or fall in the heart rate. Stroke volume isn't the only thing affecting the heart rate. So do each of the following:

- Hypoxia
- Sympathetic stimulation (pain, fear, anxiety)
- Fever (10 bpm for every degree F of temp)
- Drugs
- Exercise
- Metabolic events (myxedema coma, thyroid storm, response to injury, etc.)

You have a post-op patient with a heart rate of 110. Is this a good heart rate for this patient? Maybe. Maybe not. You can't tell without seeing the company that that number keeps. Maybe the patient came out of surgery with a heart rate of 80. That afternoon it went to 90 and the next morning it was 100. Now it is 110. What's going on? You don't know, but you do know that a climbing heart rate is the first sign of bleeding, fluid overload, hypoxia, fever, and/or metabolic events.

A climbing heart rate is your first indicator that something is going on. Sometimes devastating events occur to a patient, and later you wonder if you could have been able to see it coming before it overwhelmed you and the patient. Yes, you *can* see it coming. After a crisis, if you go back into the patient's chart, clues of the coming catastrophe can be clearly seen in the climbing heart rate. But that is hindsight. Anyone can see things in hindsight. The real skill is in seeing in real time, and your first sign of impending doom is the climbing heart rate. The acceleration in the heart rate is a compensatory mechanism. When it fails, that's when we see all those other symptoms.

Heart rate starting to climb is your first sign that patients are bleeding, getting fluid overloaded, hypoxic, or infected. This sign can only be seen by noting trends. Maybe your post-op patient came out of surgery with a heart rate of 130, the next day it was 120, and today it is 110. This patient is getting better. For every patient you have, for every number that patient generates, you must know where that number falls into that patient's continuum or you will miss the biggest subclinical sign of impending doom there is—heart rate starting to climb.

Hemodynamic Principals, Shock, and Heart Failure

Your cardiovascular system is made of your tank, your pipes, and your pump. The tank is the blood volume, the pipes are the blood vessels, and the pump is your heart.

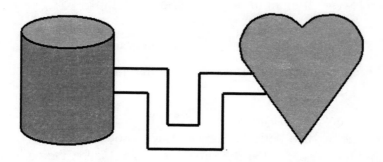

You may hear people say, *"He's two quarts low. We need to top off his tank."* They are talking about blood volume. The type of shock you get when your tank is empty is called *hypovolemic*, and it doesn't matter how you got there. I could have given you too much Lasix, you could have grabbed the stop sign. Hypovolemic is *hypovolemic*.

There are three types of shock that have to do with the pipes being too big. They are 1) *septic*—massive vasodilatation from endotoxins, 2) *anaphylactic*—massive vasodilatation from an allergic reaction, and 3) *neurogenic*—seen in patients with spinal cord injuries.

Pump failure is *cardiogenic* shock. There is a failure to fill and squeeze adequately to meet the metabolic needs of the body. This frequently causes a back up of pressure into the lungs, throwing the patient into pulmonary edema and making him hypoxic. Circulation has slowed and less oxygen is being added to the mix. This is a recipe for a lethal dysrhythmia.

These different forms of shock require different treatments. For the patient in hypovolemic shock, we must administer fluids. If the tank is empty, fill it up. For the patient with the distributive shock we can see two routes of treatment. When the pipes got bigger, the inner lumen of the vessels increased, and the fluid level in the tank dropped. Current therapy for the patient with a distributive shock is to make sure the tank is filled back up before ever adding a vasoconstrictor—the reason being that when you tighten down on someone's pipes, it greatly increases the work load of the heart, and you don't want to do that unless you absolutely have to.

For the patient in hypovolemic shock, you have fluid running lickety-split. For the patient in a distributive shock, you have fluid going lickety-split and possibly a vasoconstrictor. But what happens to the man in cardiogenic shock if we give him 4 liters of normal saline? We just killed him, didn't we? Why is the patient in cardiogenic shock so different from patients with other forms of shock?

ACUTE CONGESTIVE HEART FAILURE

The coronary arteries take off out of the cusps of the aortic valve, course across the top of the heart (where they can be bypassed) and then they turn and dive into the myocardium. When they do this, they very easily become compressed. The myocardium gets its blood supply during diastole. So the force pushing the blood down the coronary arteries is the diastolic blood pressure.

A patient called me into her room complaining of a 5/10 of her usual and accustomed chest pain. She requested a nitroglycerine tablet. Since I was a wonderful nurse, I got her blood pressure before giving it to her. She had a pressure of 110/60. Can this lady have a NTG tablet? The rule was that you could have one if there was a systolic blood pressure greater than 100 mmHg. So, I gave her the NTG tablet and within seconds we had a pressure of 70/40. A diastolic pressure of 40 mmHg was insufficient to perfuse her coronary arteries and she went into cardiogenic shock. And I went right behind her. She turned that lovely grey-green color we all hate to see in our patients, and she was waving good-bye.

When it was all over and she was stable again, I went back into her chart trying to figure out what I had done wrong. I found that her normal blood pressure was 190/100. This was in the days when we believed elderly people needed high blood pressures to perfuse their stenotic carotid arteries. We gave up on that one also. This was the first time I had ever heard the term *relative* shock. I thought shock was defined by a systolic blood pressure of > 100 mmHg. It is. It is also any time there has been more than a 40-point drop, and my patient had had an 80-point drop in her systolic pressure. She was in shock before I ever gave her the nitroglycerine tablet, and by giving it to her, I almost did her in.

When taking emergency numbers on a patient, always go back and compare those numbers to the *patient's* normal numbers, not to what *you* might think is normal. Our patients are notorious for coming into the hospital without first reading the book describing normal numbers or normal behavior. *Always* compare the emergency numbers to the patient's normal numbers or you have a set up for making big mistakes.

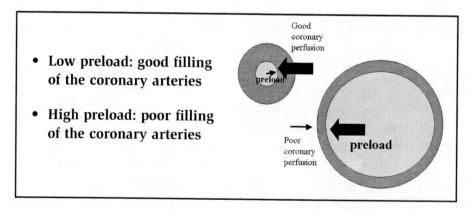

- **Low preload: good filling of the coronary arteries**

- **High preload: poor filling of the coronary arteries**

If you put a lot of blood into the heart, it stretches the walls way out. The coronary arteries still course across the top of the heart, but when they turn and dive into the myocardium, they have a heck of a time getting any blood into the muscle. The volume of blood in the heart and the pressure it puts on the walls is called the *preload*. The blood is forced down the coronary arteries by the diastolic blood pressure, but its flow is opposed by the volume of blood in the chamber and the pressure that it creates—the *preload.*

The more volume in the heart, the less able you are to perfuse the myocardium. This fluid overload state is called *congestive heart failure.* The problem in CHF is that there is too much blood in the heart, you can't get good flow down the coronary arteries, so you can't deliver oxygen to the cells for them to make ATP and run their action potentials and contract. The result is a poor squeeze in the heart with resultant pulmonary edema and hypoxia. Your patient has a lethal dysrhythmia and dies.

To treat a patient with an acute CHF, we must unload the volume and move the patient to a lesser preload so that more flow can come down the coronary arteries. To help ourselves in this endeavor we will use oxygen, Lasix, digitalis, NTG, morphine, and BNP. This is a patient with an *acute* CHF, not a chronic one, so we won't use beta blockers or ACE inhibitors.

The first thing on our list is oxygen.

I went down to the ER one day to help out because they were having "the day from hell." There were two cardiac arrests happening simultaneously and a patient having an acute MI. The novice nurse was with the MI patient, so I went to see if I could help her. I noticed that the patient didn't have any oxygen going. I asked the novice if she wanted me to put some oxygen on her patient. She replied that he didn't need it since his O_2 saturation was 97%.

What had she missed? Where do you want this oxygen? In his finger tip or in the ischemic area of his heart? Patients having cardiac problems *always* get oxygen! If the patient is a CO_2 retaining COPDer, they, more than anyone else, will need the extra oxygen to make it through the crisis. You don't just put it on and leave it on. You fix the problem and then bring down the oxygen.

I put oxygen on the patient having the MI. There was now oxygen getting into the cardiac muscle. The patient used this oxygen to make ATP to run his action potential so he didn't die of a lethal dysrhythmia, and he squeezed with it. Increased contractility equals increased stroke volume. Improved emptying drops the preload, thereby increasing flow down the coronary arteries and increasing the chances of survival.

Oxygen is an extremely benign thing to do to someone. If you had a CO_2 retaining COPDer, you might make his PCO_2 go up. *Might*. The beauty of oxygen is that you can always take it off. But remember, you squeeze with it and you run your action potential with it. So it is nice to have around, and you can always take it off.

Next on our list is Lasix. Lasix help this patient drop his preload through the elimination of extra fluid. If it is in the toilet, it's not available to come back into the heart, and the dropped preload allows more flow down the coronary arteries. Remember, you don't want to unload your patient too much, or you drop the blood pressure that forces the blood down the coronary arteries, and you still get poor myocardial perfusion. All things within moderation, please.

Digitalis helps the patient to increase myocardial contractility and thereby squeeze better and empty better. Digitalis also lowers the heart rate. Nothing consumes oxygen in the heart the way heart rate does. It gets about 85% of the available oxygen. Therefore, dropping someone's heart rate (within reason) saves oxygen that can be used to run the action potential and squeeze with.

If you give someone a nitroglycerine tablet, it causes his peripheral blood vessels to dilate and lowers his blood pressure. Blood pressure is a big part of afterload. Afterload is the amount of pressure the chamber needs to generate in order to open the valve and empty its contents.

Therefore, the first part of afterload to consider is the quality of the valve in question. If the valve leaflets are just little tissue paper things that easily lay back against the aorta—the way they should—it doesn't take much energy to move them. But if the valve leaflets are stuck together and you have to push pretty hard to open them, or if you have a tight stenotic opening that you are trying to cram all the blood through, that will require even more energy, and the value for afterload goes up.

Once you get the valve open, blood pressure is a very large component of afterload, but consider also the consistency of the blood and compliance of the blood vessels. It is harder to shove around sludge than it is to shove around fruit punch. Your patient's hematocrit is a part of his afterload as is the compliance of the blood vessels. If the vessels are young and healthy, they easily bulge out with each bolus of blood. Not much energy is required. But if you have tough, old blood vessels, or if you have a vasoconstrictor on the outside of the blood vessels, it will increase the work load for the heart. The afterload goes up.

Our next treatment for the acute CHF patient is morphine. In this instance, morphine is not for pain; it is there to decrease the circulating catecholamines. The catecholamines are the neurotransmitters for the sympathetic nervous system that make the heart rate and blood pressure go up. If the heart rate and blood pressure don't go up, you save oxygen that can be used to run the action potential and squeeze with.

Decreasing circulating catecholamines can be done with a Valium tablet. The problem is that Valium takes forever to get into the blood stream and forever to get back out. You want something that is fast-acting and quickly metabolized if you decide that you no longer want it around. Morphine fits that bill. Some doctors are switching to Dilaudid for the same reasons. Although we don't always know what we are doing, medicine is often a matter of opinion. You should always do what works best for this particular patient.

BNP (Natrecor) is a new treatment on the market for congestive heart failure. It is both a treatment and a diagnostic tool. Sometimes it is difficult to determine whether a patient is having an MI or is in congestive heart failure, and you need to know as treatments vary. Measuring serum BNP levels can tell you. The numbers are elevated in patients with CHF. If you have CHF, the clinician can infuse BNP into the patient, often with dramatic improvement. The action of BNP is uncertain, but it has been shown to lower pulmonary artery wedge pressure better than nitroglycerine, probably by vasodilation.

Cardiac Output

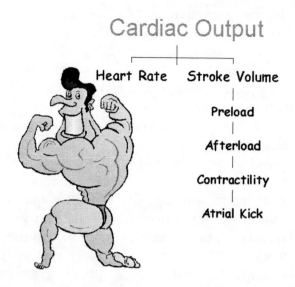

Heart Rate   Stroke Volume

Preload

Afterload

Contractility

Atrial Kick

Cardiac output is heart rate times stroke volume. Heart rate is a factor of sympathetic/parasympathetic innervation into the SA node. Stroke volume has several components. The first is preload. You can't get out what you didn't put in. Afterload is resistance to flow—the higher it is, the less well the heart empties. Contractility—how hard did you squeeze, and did you get your atrial kick —signified by one 'p' in front of every "QRS." These are the components of stroke volume.

If you give someone a cardiac medication, you do it to improve his cardiac output by manipulating any of the above factors. By the same token, if your patient has a problem in any of these areas, it negatively effects cardiac output and you need to get it fixed.

SYMPTOMS OF LEFT AND RIGHT HEART FAILURE

We are forever showing students diagrams of the cardiovascular system that make you think that the right heart looks the same as the left heart. They don't look anything like each other. If you took a heart (turkey and beef are good, chicken a little hard to see, and human not recommended), cut it in half, and turned it on its side, in the center you would see an inconstant inner lumen of the left ventricle and a large muscle mass around it. To the outside of the large muscle mass there is a slit with a thin muscle mass around it. This is the right ventricle.

The right ventricle literally wraps around the left ventricle. They don't look anything like each other while having the same volumes. But we teachers are forever showing you diagrams that make you think they do—like the following one.

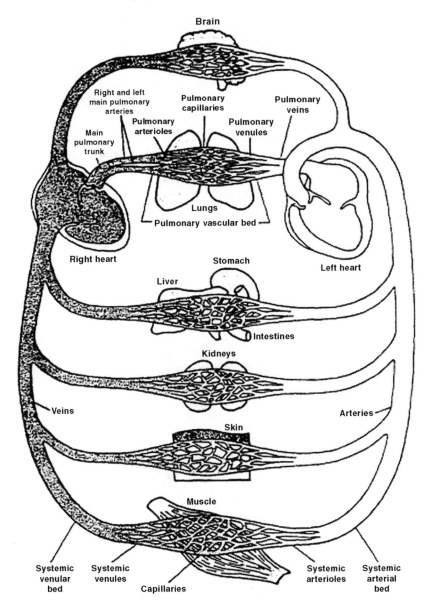

Next we are going to look at right and left heart failure. I know it is possible to ruin your right heart with your left heart, and vice versa, and that people do it all the time. But for the purposes of this teaching example we will look at pure right and pure left heart failure.

The deoxygenated blood leaves the right heart and goes to the lungs where the RBCs are saturated to the best of their ability with oxygen. The blood then goes to the left ventricle where it is pumped out into the systemic circulation where the oxygen and other good things are delivered to the cells. The deoxygenated blood then comes back into the right heart where it is pumped into the lungs, and the journey begins again.

Around and around it goes in a clockwise—and only clockwise—fashion. Because the blood moves only in a clockwise fashion, should you obstruct the blood flow, you will see the pressure begin to increase downstream from the trouble.

RIGHT HEART FAILURE

We will begin first with right heart failure. There are numerous things that can cause your right heart to fail. You can infarct it, get a myopathy, or one very efficient way to make it fail is for the pressure in the lungs to go up. The thin-walled right ventricle cannot push against high pressures, and it fails. *Cor pulmonale* is right heart failure secondary to *pulmonary hypertension*. For whatever reason, we now have right heart failure.

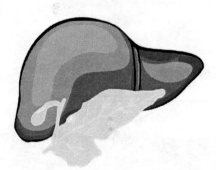

Because the blood cannot flow smoothly through the right heart, pressure begins to back up downstream. One of the first places you see a problem is in the liver. The liver becomes engorged and enlarges. We say the liver drops because it can be easily felt down in the abdomen. The liver is responsible for the metabolism of fats, carbohydrates, and protein. It makes precursors to hormones, clotting factors, and is a huge filter. None of this is going to work well when it is engorged.

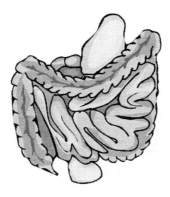

The guts also become engorged as the walls swell from the increased pressure. Nutrition is crucial for keeping your patient alive, but they are supposed to absorb the nutrients through the microvillus in the small intestine, and these are swollen closed. Right heart failure patients have lots of digestive and nutrition problems.

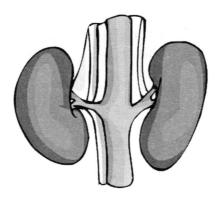

Urine is made in the kidneys by a pure pressure-driven system. If the pressure distal to the kidney goes up, the amount of urine being made goes down. Besides urine production, the kidneys are responsible for balancing pH, electrolytes, fluid, and removing waste products.

All are things that, if not done right, can make you dead. Kidney function is very important to health and well being.

The pressure also backs up into the skin, making these patients have edematous extremities. Blood flows through the muscles dropping off oxygen to make ATP to exercise with. If the pressure distal goes up, flow goes down, and exercise capacity drops off.

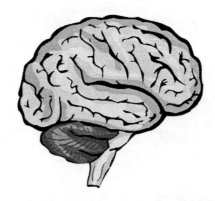

The brain is also trying to send blood back into the right heart, and it also becomes edematous and you get a change in mentation. Everything in life occurs along a continuum. At one end of the mentation continuum, patients are obtunded and unresponsive to pain. At the other end of the continuum the signs may be so subtle you can hardly perceive them.

It can be as subtle as a change in personality. You have a patient who has been a sweetheart who is now a bear. Take a look at his I & O. Nine times out of ten, he's getting fluid overloaded. For women, once a month the world goes out of whack. We stay the same, the world gets weird. We think what happens is that we retain a bunch of fluid that gives us a touch of cerebral edema, and irritability is a sign of the cerebral edema. If you have a patient who appears suddenly irritable, check the I & O before getting involved in a confrontation.

Did you have to tell a patient something only once yesterday, but have had to tell him twice today? That may be another early sign of change in mentation. Or maybe you are in the patient's room walking around, and he isn't paying any attention to you. If someone was walking around your bedroom would you be paying attention? Of course you would. If that person is known to carry enema tubes and needles in her hands, you are paying *close* attention! If you speak to a patient, she may answer appropriately, and then just drift away. This could be another early sign of change in mentation.

You have a patient with a pure right heart failure. You cannot hear rales in the lungs. Why not? The lungs are not downstream from the right heart. Let's give our patient left heart failure. Can you hear rales in the lungs of patients with a pure left heart failure? Yes, because the lungs are now downstream.

It is now time to look at the continuum of respiratory distress. At the far end of the continuum, the patient just had a hypoxic code and died of a lethal dysrhythmia. But the very first sign of respiratory distress is very subtle. The only energy source in the human body is ATP which is made of oxygen and glucose. Keeping the amount of oxygen in the bloodstream normal is crucial to keeping us alive. If the amount of oxygen in the bloodstream was dropping off, the first thing you would do to get it back up again is to breathe faster.

Your very first sign of respiratory distress is that the patient has increased his respiratory rate. All other numbers are the same. The patient was breathing 12 times a minute yesterday and had an O_2 saturation of 95%. Today, he is breathing 22 times a minute and has an O_2 saturation of 95%. Is there a change? Your subclinical sign of respiratory distress is that the patient has increased his respiratory rate. When increasing the respiratory rate *fails* to alleviate the problem, all the *clinical* signs begin.

If a patient is going into congestive heart failure, before he pours a lot of fluid into the alveolar space where you can hear it as rales, the first thing he does is to swell up his interstitium. The interstitium is the space between the capillary and the alveolar lumen that the oxygen needs to diffuse across. When the distance between the alveoli and the capillary becomes greater, the amount of oxygen making it into the circulation goes down, and in response, the respiratory rate goes up. Your very first sign of congestive heart failure is that the patient's respiratory rate has simply picked up. The shortness of breath, rales in the lungs, and bad O_2 sats all come after this compensatory mechanism has failed. The better the patient's compensatory mechanisms, the longer he will maintain himself by breathing faster.

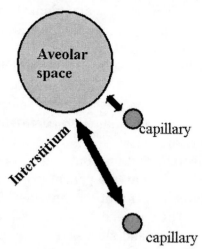

When studying post-op patients that were so overloaded with fluid that they ended up in the intensive care unit, it could be determined from the patient's chart the exact shift during which they went into failure. But that is hindsight. The really hard thing to do is to see it in real time. The subclinical signs are the respiratory rate and heart rate beginning to climb and the urine output beginning to drop off—not to become abnormally low, but to be less than it had been.

We just looked at why the respiratory rate began to climb, let's move back into the heart and see why the heart rate began to climb, and then later into the kidneys to see why the urine output drops off.

Cardiac output is heart rate times stroke volume. With our left heart failure we have developed poor squeeze from any one of many reasons. The heart does not squeeze as well as it used to, and stroke volume goes down. To compensate, heart rate goes up. This is why the heart rate goes up in the patient with left heart failure.

The heart is now squeezing less well, and heart rate has picked up to attempt to keep the cardiac output adequate to meet the body's metabolic needs. The purpose of the left heart is to pump the oxygenated blood into the systemic circulation and out to the cells. In order to achieve this, the perfusion pressure must stay high enough, but we have poor squeeze and the pressures have dropped off. In order to compensate for this we vasoconstrict.

Once the blood vessels are vasoconstricted, blood pressure is no longer a good indicator of how the patient is doing. If the blood pressure is low, indeed you do have a problem, but don't be fooled into thinking everything is OK because the pressure is normal or high. If you have a vasoconstricted patient, blood pressure is not a good indicator of how they are doing, but heart rate is. Heart rate is a direct look into the patient's heart at how well it is squeezing (contractility). If the heart is squeezing well, stroke volume goes up. To compensate for the increased volume, heart rate goes down. Squeeze less well, heart rate goes up in an attempt to keep the total volume constant.

The patient in left heart failure is frequently vasoconstricted throughout the body. Vasoconstrict into the brain and you get the same change of mentation anywhere along the continuum. Vasoconstrict into the liver and it doesn't work any better than it did all engorged. Vasoconstrict into the guts and you can have very serious problems.

Inside our digestive system we have some very caustic substances, such as hydrochloric acid and pancreatic enzymes, that are there to help us digest our food. These are non-selective digesters. They would be just as happy to digest *us* at the same time. To protect us from this unfortunate (and painful) event, we have a wonderful gastric mucosa. It must be repaired constantly, using the food we eat, that comes via the circulatory system, and using ATP as an energy source. If there is decreased blood flow into the gut, we do not repair as well as we should. It is also possible to infarct and make ulcers.

Our digestive system is filled with bacteria. They are our friends. We want them there. But, we want them there under *our* conditions. One of those conditions is that the colony counts must stay down. To keep the colony counts down, every day or so we deposit multitudes of them into the toilet and flush them away. This requires peristalsis, which requires muscle contraction, which requires blood flow, ATP, etc. Decreased blood flow into the gut decreases peristalsis, which allows the bacteria to live long, reproduce constantly, and pump all kinds of toxins into the patient, making her feel awful. Left heart failure patients have *lots* of GI distress.

Vasoconstrict into the kidneys and they still don't make urine. This is why urine output begins to drop off in the acute CHF patient. If you vasoconstrict into the muscles, less oxygen is delivered, less ATP made, and exercise capacity goes down. Vasoconstrict into the skin and we get cold, clammy, diaphoretic skin. We now know that diaphoresis is a very ominous sign. It is a sympathetic response that uses a parasympathetic neurotransmitter. That's nice, but why should you care? Because any patient that is diaphoretic is maximally sympathetically stimulated. They are using everything they have to keep those numbers right where they are.

Along with being a very ominous sign, it is also a very *distinctive* sign. Once you have seen it, felt it, and someone has told you what you are looking at, you will never miss it again. But having someone tell you what you are looking at is the key to learning. One of the things that we don't do well today is that we don't mentor young nurses around us very well. In the good old days when you came out of nursing school, you were the most pathetic thing who ever graduated. But, when you came to the hospital floor there were all these nurses around, and one of them took pity on you and taught you to be a nurse.

Today when you come out of nursing school, you are still the most pathetic thing to ever walk across the stage, but when you reach the nursing floor there aren't all those nurses to help you learn to be a nurse. You have one nurse running up and down the hallway as fast as he can and another nurse running up and down the other hallway as fast as she can. They don't even *talk* to each other, much less mentor each other. We are losing tremendous amounts of nursing knowledge because we don't think we have the time to pass it on.

There is about to be a crisis in the nursing profession like no other crisis we have seen. The crisis is our aging work force. About 60% of the nurses working in 2004 were in their early 50s and older. The really, *really* big problem is that if the stock market ever goes up again, the baby-boomer nurses are all retiring. Potentially 60% of the nursing work force will be retiring in the next ten years or so. And which is the next group that is going to need large quantities of nursing care? Us old nurses! The government has already recognized that a lack of nursing care is one of the problems that retired baby boomers will face. So many of the baby boomers were nurses themselves, and fewer people are entering the profession. Please take the time to mentor the young nurses around you!

Non-invasive Signs of Poor Cardiac Output

We have been looking at the non-invasive signs of poor cardiac output. These are things you can see without sending the patient to the diagnostic center and without having a million dollar machine come to the bedside. These signs are:

1. change in mentation, anywhere along the continuum,
2. respiratory distress, anywhere along the continuum,
3. the heart rate is up,
4. the liver is engorged,
5. GI problems have increased,
6. urine output has dropped off,
7. the skin is edematous and/or cold, clammy, and diaphoretic, and
8. exercise capacity has decreased.

If you are working with a patient in an acute situation, and you want to know how well you are oxygenating and perfusing the patient's cells, there are three good indicators. They don't come in any order; they frequently come all at once. They are 1) a change in mentation, because neurons are so sensitive to hypoxia; 2) rate of ectopy (irregular heart beats) because the action potential is so sensitive to hypoxia, and 3) diaphoresis because it shows maximal sympathetic stimulation. Any of these getting better—nice work! Any of these getting worse—work harder! If the patient flutters his eyes open and looks at you—*yahoo!* If he rolls his back in his head—*work harder!*

In the long run, if you want to know how well a patient is doing, the improvement can be measured in exercise capacity. If a patient has come to you to get better, he should be better every single day, and it can be seen in an improvement in exercise capacity. How do you know if a patient is increasing his exercise capacity? You have to have concrete markers that all staff recognize. In one hospital they have 25 foot markers on the wall, so they can say the patient went 25 feet, 100 feet, 350 feet. They are all talking the same language.

What do you mean when you say the patient ambulated well? What I mean is that the patient had no signs of poor cardiac output during the time he was being ambulated. That is a nurse's decision to make, not a nurse's aide's. In an ideal situation, you and the aide would ambulate the patient together, but we seldom get ideal. The least I want you to settle for is being able to watch it happen. Tell the aide that when she is going to ambulate the patient, she should let you know. Then make sure you watch it happen, because whether or not the patient ambulated well is *your* decision.

If a patient needs oxygen to lay in bed, she needs oxygen to walk down the hall. Nurse's aides do not understand this. In their two weeks of nursing school, ATP formation and action potentials never came up once. If you are going to increase your patient's exercise level, she needs her oxygen. If you deny the patient her oxygen, your walk will turn into a drag. There will be two or more of you dragging the hypoxic patient back to bed.

We are forever assigning knowledge to nurse's aides that they do not have. Because they do their chores well, we think they understand the reason behind their actions, and often they don't. They are simply repeating actions without understanding underlying causes or treatment goals. It is the *nurse* who possesses this knowledge. It is the *nurse* who needs to guide the aide; the *nurse* who understands the why.

Time for a quick quiz:

What are the things that make you heart rate go up?

ANSWER: Stroke volume falling because you are under or overloaded, hypoxia, fever, sympathetic stimulation (pain, fear, anxiety), exercise, drugs.

What are things that make your respiratory rate go up?

ANSWER: Hypoxia, metabolic acidosis, sympathetic stimulation, exercise, psychological factors

Always confirm that the patient is not hypoxic before reaching for the Ativan! Hypoxia makes you very anxious and if the people around you are saying stupid things like, "Slow your breathing down," or "Just relax," it is pretty easy to come unglued, because you know you are having a life-threatening event, and you can't get anyone to believe you!

Metabolic acidosis will also increase the respiratory rate as the patient tries to compensate for the lactic acidosis he is experiencing by blowing off CO_2 in an attempt to bring the pH back to normal by picking up his respiratory rate. If you ever have a patient breathing too fast for no apparent respiratory reason, ask yourself whether or not it might be compensation for lactic acidosis.

I was asked to see a patient in the diagnostic center that had just had another set of bilateral nephrostomy tubes replaced. The radiology tech called and said, *"I don't know what is wrong with him. He just doesn't look right. Would you come see him?"* I told him I would be right there. When I arrived the patient was lying on the gurney with his head elevated 45 degrees. His blood pressure and heart rate were slightly elevated, and he was somewhat flushed, but placing nephrostomy tubes is hard, painful work. He was also breathing rapidly. Being the excellent nurse that I am, I felt this was something that needed to be followed up on. I whipped out my stethoscope and placed it on his chest. I clearly heard normal breath sounds throughout both lung fields. I asked him if he was short of breath, and he said, *"No."* I asked, *"Then why are you breathing so fast?"* and he said, *"I don't know."* Within 30 minutes he was in the ICU, on a ventilator, and in septic shock. The increased in respiration was his attempt to compensation for the lactic acidosis being caused by his sepsis.

He must have had a pocket of some very virulent organisms left over from another set of tubes, and when they placed these new tubes, they must have gone right through it, spreading the organisms throughout his body. If you ever have a patient breathing too fast for no apparent reason, ask yourself whether it might be compensation of a metabolic acidosis—and in our work environment, sepsis is a likely candidate.

Two other things that can make your respiratory rate go up are exercise and sympathetic stimulation. Another cause for an increase in respiration is anxiety. I have a very hard time with the psychological diagnosis being given because the most likely recipient of that label is a woman.

WOMEN'S HEART DISEASE

As recently as the 1970s, if a woman complained to her doctor of chest pain, her doctor's likely diagnosis was anxiety. Heart disease was assumed to be a male disease. Women who complained of chest pain were assumed to be women who wanted to be men, and it manifested itself in this bizarre need to have a male disease. A doctor may have prescribed Valium for this poor woman and sent her off to see a psychiatrist where she could discuss her gender identity issues.

Well, women *do* have heart disease. It is the number one killer of women over age 45. So, maybe these women didn't have gender identity issues; maybe they had myocardial ischemia.

Several years ago, drug companies got into trouble with the US government because they had not included women in their cardiac drug studies. Why not? Women are in diabetes, arthritis, and numerous other studies; why aren't they in the cardiac studies? They started out being in the cardiac studies, but it skewed the results. The data didn't make any sense any more. Since it was assumed that women didn't *have* heart disease, drug companies excluded them from the studies, and then the data made perfect sense. (The good news is that the discarded Framingham data on women still exists for study)

The following data is from the National Center for Health Statistics; National Heart, Lung, and Blood Institute, and the American Heart Association, and is published on the National Coalition for Women with Heart Disease web site (www.womenheart.org).

Prevalence

- 8,000,000 American women are currently living with heart disease—10% of women ages 45–64 and 25% age 65 and over.
- 6,000,000 of women today have a history of heart attack and/or angina or both.
- Nearly 13% of women age 45 and over have had a heart attack.

- 435,000 American women have heart attacks each year; 83,000 are under age 65 and 9,000 are under age 45. Their average age is 70.4.
- 4,000,000 women suffer from angina, and 47,000 of them were hospitalized in 1999.

Mortality

- Heart disease is the leading cause of death of American women and kills 32% of them.
- 43% of deaths in American women, or nearly 500,000, are caused by cardiovascular disease (heart disease and stroke) each year.
- 267,000 women die each year from heart attacks, which kill six times as many women as breast cancer.
- 31,837 women die each year of congestive heart failure, or 62.6% of all heart failure deaths.

At-Risk

- The age-adjusted rate of heart disease for African American women is 72% higher than for white women, while African American women ages 55–64 are twice as likely as white women to have a heart attack and 35% more likely to suffer from coronary artery disease.
- Women who smoke risk having a heart attack 19 years earlier than non-smoking women.
- Women with diabetes are two to three times more likely to have heart attacks.
- High blood pressure is more common in women taking oral contraceptives, especially in obese women.
- 39% of white women, 57% of black women, 57% of Hispanic women, and 49% Asian/Pacific Islander women are sedentary and get no leisure time physical activity.
- 23% of white women, 38% of black women, and 36% Mexican American women are obese.

Compared with Men

- 38% of women and 25% of men will die within one year of a first recognized heart attack.

- 35% of women and 18% of men heart attack survivors will have another heart attack within six years.

- 46% of women and 22% of men heart attack survivors will be disabled with heart failure within six years.

- Women are almost twice as likely as men to die after bypass surgery.

- Women are less likely than men to receive beta-blockers, ACE inhibitors or even aspirin after a heart attack.

- More women than men die of heart disease each year, yet women receive only:

   33% of angioplasties, stents and bypass surgeries

   28% of implantable defibrillators and

   36% of open-heart surgeries

- Women comprise only 25% of participants in all heart-related research studies.

Women *do* have heart disease. Does it matter that the cardiac studies were done on men? Women just have smaller hearts, don't they? No, they don't. There is fascinating research coming out right now on the structural and functional differences between male and female members of the species. Not only are our brains structurally different, our hearts function differently. Let's look at one way in which male and female hearts differ from each other.

This representation was replicated in the study *Gender related differences in cardiac response to supine exercise assessed by radionuclide angiography,* published in the *American Journal of Cardiology 13(3), 624–9* on March 1, 1989.

The numbers in the depictions are totally arbitrary and are meant for illustrative purposes only.

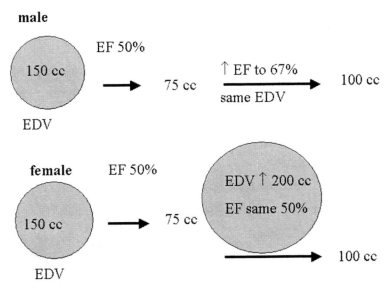

We will look first at the male heart because that is the model. The volume in the heart at the end of diastole is called the end diastolic volume (EDV). It included passive filling and the artial kick. Let's place 150cc of blood into the heart with an ejection fraction (EF) of 50%, which means that every time the heart squeezes, half of the EDV is ejected, or 75cc of blood. The 75cc is called the stroke volume. Later, the man needs to increase his stroke volume to 100cc with each beat (or stroke) of his heart. What the man does is to increase his ejection fraction to about 67%. He squeezes harder on the same 150cc of blood and gets out 100cc.

Next, let's watch the woman do it. We will give her the same starting numbers as the man—EDV 150cc, EF 50% and a stroke volume of 75cc. The woman now needs to increase her output with each beat to 100cc—maybe she is exercising or has just seen Mel Gibson walk past. The woman does not increase her ejection fraction. She increases her EDV (total volume in the heart) to 200cc, squeezes with the same 50% ejection fraction, and gets out 100cc.

The man and woman have gotten the same end result, but by two totally different pathways. It would not matter that they did it differently unless most of your tests that looked for myocardial ischemia were based on changes in ejection fraction. If you were looking for changes in ejection fraction in women, you would not see it.

A woman having her first MI is statistically much more likely to die from it than a man. One reason could be that it is not picked up before she has *The Big One*. Part of the problem is the way we teach people about angina. We used to teach it based on the male model. We said angina feels like an elephant sitting on your chest or a band around your heart. It radiates down your arm, into your back, or up your jaw. Well, it does if you are a man, but a woman having symptoms of myocardial ischemia can present very differently.

Signs of Female Myocardial Ischemia

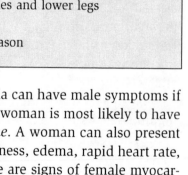

Angina — tightness in the chest, sometimes radiating down left arm or into the jaw. Often mistaken for indigestion.

Breathlessness — chronic or nocturnal dyspnea

Chronic fatigue — usually overwhelming

Dizziness — unexplained lightheadedness, even blackouts

Edema — swelling, particularly of the ankles and lower legs

Fluttering or rapid heartbeat

Gastric upset — nausea for no apparent reason

A woman having myocardial ischemia can have male symptoms if she wants to. One study I read said that a woman is most likely to have male symptoms when she has *The Big One*. A woman can also present with breathlessness, chronic fatigue, dizziness, edema, rapid heart rate, and nausea for no apparent reason. These are signs of female myocardial ischemia, and they are misdiagnosed all the time. Women who have been diagnosed with chronic fatigue syndrome have been found to actually have myocardial ischemia.

The signs of female myocardial ischemia are sometimes very vague and very difficult to pick up. However, we have known for well over a decade that women having myocardial ischemia present differently from men. Surely, no woman relaying the above symptoms to her doctor would miss a cardiac work-up today. *Right?* Wrong. It happens all the time.

Joyce was a 53-year-old head nurse of a telemetry floor. For 2 years she had been going to her family physician complaining of these exact symptoms. Every time she came back from seeing her doctor, she had a new drug. He had given her Zoloft since she appeared depressed and Xanax for her anxiety attacks. She had hydrochlorthiazide for the swelling in her ankles and something for her tummy. The last time she saw him he gave her pills to help her loose weight.

Two years into this, Joyce goes to work one day feeling that something is just *wrong* inside. Because of this, she put on a telemetry pack and wore it all day which nearly gave the telemetry tech a stroke. She had by far the worst-looking heart of any patient admitted to the floor that day. She had a left bundle branch block, (which implies a tremendous amount of muscle damage), polymorphic PVCs, and runs of Vtach.

She took her telemetry strips back to her family practice doc and said, "I want a cardiac work-up!" The doc was not impressed, feeling that most of it could be explained away by stress, anxiety, and too much caffeine intake. But he relented, and Joyce got her cardiac work-up. She was found to have cardiomyopathy with an ejection fraction of 10%. That meant that each time her heart contracted, only 10% of the total volume came out, leaving 90% behind in the heart.

Now, how in the world are you taking care of patients with an ejection fraction of 10%? How do you compensate for such a disaster? You do it by having a huge heart. If you had a heart with 100cc in it with an ejection fraction of 10%, how much would come out each time it contracted? You would get 10cc. That simply won't do. But what if you had a heart with 1000 cc in it, how much would you get out with your 10% ejection fraction? 100cc. Joyce actually had a normal cardiac output, but she did it by having a *huge* heart!

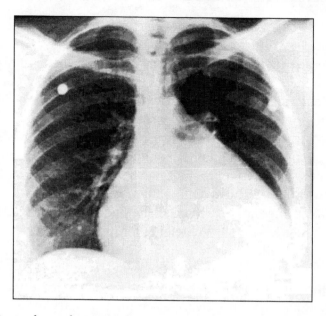

Having a huge heart is the compensatory mechanism, but this is fraught with problems. The big heart crowds out the lungs and there goes exercise capacity. Valve leaflets get pulled apart, allowing for mitral valve regurgitation which leads to pulmonary hypertension. The walls of the heart are stretched thin and you cannot get good blood flow into the myocardium to deliver oxygen to make ATP to squeeze and run the action potential. Patients with enlarged hearts develop what is technically called "crappy squeeze" (systolic heart failure) and since they cannot repolarize their action potential, a lethal dysrhythmia is a frequent mode of passing on to the next reality.

You don't usually get a 1000cc heart. There is no room for it in the chest. You get a 500cc heart that beats twice as fast as anyone else's. Joyce had a resting heart rate of 120 beats per minute. I don't know what the doctor thought of that. Maybe he thought she was just happy to see him, or maybe that she was having an anxiety attack. He never took the chest X-ray that would have shown the huge heart and never did an EKG that would have shown the myocardial damage.

Once Joyce got her diagnosis, the docs were very happy to give us old nurses cardiac work-ups. Most of us did just fine. However, the woman who was the head of the ER had been complaining of the classic signs of female myocardial ischemia for a year. Her doctor had told her, *"Look, you have a very stressful life. You are the director of the ER and your mother with Alzheimer's lives with you. Here, take this Zoloft, try to relax, and you could stand to loose a little weight."* She got her cardiac work-up and she had a high proximal LAD stenosis. The left anterior artery feeds the main pumping chamber of the heart. If you infarct it without collateral arteries to take over, you are dead. She now has a lovely stent in place and she will live a long and healthy life. So, yes you can have a stressful life, be overweight, *and* have heart disease.

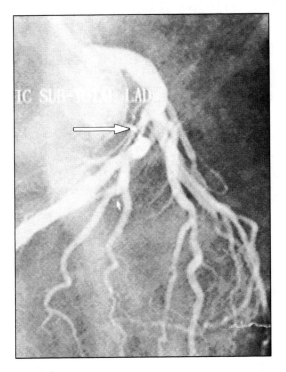

Heart disease is the number one killer of women over 45 years of age. More than all the cancers combined, cardiovascular disease is what kills women, and it is constantly misdiagnosed. In a 1999–2001 National Heart, Lung and Blood Institute and American Heart Association study of 647 post-MI women, they found the most common symptoms the women experienced before they had their MI to be fatigue, sleep disturbance, shortness of breath, indigestion, anxiety, appetite changes, aching arms, and frequent headaches.

Women present so differently from men, and female myocardial ischemia is missed so frequently. Doctors are becoming more aware of 70 to 80-year-old women having MIs, but they are less tuned in to women in their 50s having MIs, and they frequently miss *young* women with heart disease. I have a friend whose mother had her *first* MI when she was 35. Women can have heart disease early just like men can have it early in life. 435,000 women have heart attacks each year. Of these, 83,000 are under age 65, and 9,000 less that 45 years old.

Because women present so differently, they are going to need to drive the system themselves. If you feel that you may have heart disease and your family practice doctor won't give you a cardiac work-up—change doctors. More than anything else, it is cardiovascular disease that kills women, and it is missed all the time.

Adult Respiratory Distress Syndrome (ARDS)

6

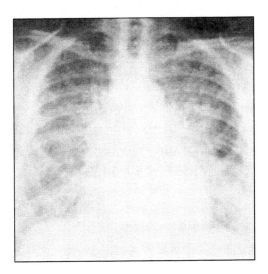

A dult Respiratory Distress Syndrome is a devastating thing to have happen to your patient. Whether your patient will survive depends on the patient's resources going into the event, the severity of the causative agent, and whether or not the event has been curtailed. Overriding these three factors is how long things went undetected and untreated. A key to surviving ARDS is early detection and treatment, frequently requiring an ICU bed and a ventilator.

Before we can delve into what goes wrong in ARDS, we need to study the inflammatory process. When people speak of the response to injury, they are talking about inflammation. The inflammatory process is what the body uses to clean up debris, heal wounds, make scars, and reestablish functioning. It is also the body's response to injury. Imagine that your skin was punctured by a thorn. When the thorn came into the skin it damaged cells and brought in bacteria. The damaged cells need to be removed, the bacteria eliminated, and the skin repaired. It is the inflammatory process that will do this for us.

The general in the battle against the invaders is a roving T cell. The T cell senses the problem and begins to call for his warriors—the white cells in the blood stream. The vast majority of the white cells in your body are not floating around where you can count them with a CBC, they are marginated—clinging to the walls of the blood vessel. This is how you can have a normal white count one day and 20,000 the next day. You didn't have to make the white cells overnight, they were already there, kind of like in suspended animation, which is a really neat way to keep your warriors.

The T cell will secrete a series of chemical mediators to make the parts of the inflammatory process happen. One of the first mediators secreted is a signal to the blood vessel to vasodilate. You want more blood with more white cells to mount the attack. The T cell then sends a signal to the marginated white cells and tells them to demarginate, get ready to go. If all they did was drop off the wall, they would be washed away, but they actually get kind of sticky and stay where the need is.

INCREASED CAPILLARY PERMEABILITY

Now, this is all really nice, but it is happening inside the blood vessel and our problem is outside the blood vessel. Luckily, our blood vessels are not lead pipes; they have slit pores that you can open up. If those pores opened up big enough to let something as big as a white cell out, do you suppose some plasma might leak out also? Of course it does.

The capillary pores are open and the white cells are out, but they don't know where to go. However, the T cell has laid down a chemotaxic smell trail. The white cells smell their way up to the problem. When they get there, they begin to secrete proteases that destroy protein, so they can clean up the debris of torn cells and begin to phago-cytize the bacteria. The white blood cells know what to get, because the T cell marks things for them. It puts a tag on the bad guys saying, *"Get this."*

This is the inflammatory process. The physical signs of inflammation reflect the pathophysiology going on. The redness and heat come from vasodilation, the swelling from increased capillary permeability, and the exudate from the white cell attack on the bacteria. Pain is a way of getting the macro individuals attention to the problem so that maybe she will pluck the thorn out and aid the healing process. The pain is generated by pressure on the nerves from the swelling and by direct irritation of the nerves by chemical mediators secreted by the T cell.

This is the inflammatory process. It is a delightful process that is meant to be kept localized. If you take it and spread it throughout your entire body, it is called Systemic Inflammatory Response Syndrome (SIRS) and it is a very bad idea.

We had never had a patient with SIRS, or it's respiratory component ARDS, until we invented the ventilator. Anyone going into SIRS or ARDS before there were ventilators would have died and we would never have seen it. But because we *did* invent ventilators, we had a way of keeping people alive past the point that they ordinarily would have died, and we can see all kinds of normal compensatory mechanisms running amok in the patient's body.

The first time we noticed this problem was during the Vietnam war. It was the first time we had ventilators on a large number of people in one area. You took a healthy male who suffered a severe trauma and placed him on a ventilator. He did okay for a few days, and then all of a sudden he got a severe hypoxia, a white out on his chest x-ray, and he died despite the most heroic efforts of the medical staff. We originally called it Da Nang lung, shock lung, or white lung. Years later, we said this is adult respiratory distress syndrome.

We also noticed that these patients tended to have cascading organ failure occurring at the same time. Originally, we said that it was most unfortunate, but it just happened. Years later, we determined that the organ failure and respiratory failure were of common origin—SIRS. SIRS hits every organ system in the body at the same time. ARDS is the respiratory component, disseminated intravascular coagulaopathy (DIC) is the hematological component, acute renal failure (ARF) is the renal component, liver failure (LF) in all its forms is the hepatic component, and having low blood pressure is the cardiovascular component. It hits the body all at once, but most often you see it in the lungs first.

The different components of SIRS are all tied together so that if you get one you are at risk for all the others. For example, lets suppose that you are a fireman who inhales smoke at a fire and gets ARDS. Now that you have ARDS, you are at risk for renal failure, DIC, liver failure, and cardiovascular collapse. Anyone having any of the component parts of SIRS, places himself into SIRS, and is at risk for all the other entities involved. Being in shock places you at risk for liver failure, renal failure, DIC, etc.

Who is at Risk to go into ARDS?

- Shock
- Sepsis
- Trauma
- Lung contusion
- Diffuse infectious pneumonia
- Aspiration

- Heart-lung bypass
- Near drowning
- Surface burns
- Oxygen toxicity
- Pancreatitis
- Fat embolus
- DIC

If survival depends on early detection, who is at risk to go into SIRS and ARDS? Anyone who has been in shock for any reason at all, including cardiac syncope patients, septic patients, trauma patients (and the more bones you break the more likely you are to go into SIRS) people with lung contusions (those are people with seat belt abrasions), people who have had CPR, or who have been hit, kicked, or landed on their chests, people with a diffuse infectious pneumonia (SARS is a diffuse infectious pneumonia), and aspiration patients (and if they don't get ARDS, they get aspiration pneumonitis and dissolve their own lung tissue, which is not a better deal).

Anyone who has been on heart lung bypass is at risk. Your body never intended to have its blood sucked out of it in a plastic tube and then put back in again. It considers that an injury and sets off the response to injury—inflammation. This is one reason there is such an interest in doing open heart surgery on a beating heart and avoiding bypass altogether. People with surface burns are at risk, and of course the more burn the more risk. If you survived your near-drowning and now have respiratory distress, it is frequently ARDS. Oxygen toxicity kills via the ARDS pathway.

Those with pancreatitis are at risk because "itis" means inflammation. Any disease ending in "itis," if sent systemic, can result in SIRS and ARDS. I had a patient who did it with myocarditis. DIC patients are at risk for ARDS because DIC is the hematological component of SIRS, and having one component opens you up to all of them. Patients with a fat embolus are also at risk. These are the risk factors for going into ARDS and of course the severity of the symptoms, the patient's reserves, and the virility of the causative agent are key to determining patient outcome.

Pathophysiology of ARDS

- Initial insult (via blood or airway)
- Set off the response to injury—inflammatory mediators
- Oxygen radicals attack cell membranes
- Proteases destroy collagen and elastin
- Capillary pores open and are stuck open

What happens physiologically with ARDS? First, you have an insult to the system setting off the response to injury. Out come the mediators, the capillaries dilate (there goes the blood pressure), oxygen radicals attack cell membranes, proteases destroy collagen and elastin (things you don't necessarily want destroyed), capillary permeability increases, and fluid pours out of the capillaries. There goes what little blood pressure you had left, and the lungs eventually fill with fluid. The causative problem in SIRS and ARDS is that the capillary permeability increases, the pores open up, and are stuck open so that only some of the fluid you give them stays contained within the cardiovascular system.

THE CLINICAL PICTURE OF ARDS

The key to patient survival is early detection. Where do people go into ARDS? On the hospital floor in the middle of the night. Or they come into clinics and ERs with it. Or they are discharged too soon into extended care facilities with it. They can also come into ICUs ARDS subtly present or with a full blown crisis. It is the continuum thing again. If you are supposed to detect it, what does it look like?

- Severe, acute, rapid onset of life threatening hypoxia
- Impaired oxygenation refractory to O_2 therapy
- Breath sounds unremarkable
- SOB with respiratory alkalosis
- Tachycardia
- Agitation

It is a severe, acute onset of life-threatening hypoxia that oxygen does not make better. By severe, acute onset, I don't mean that it is like blowing a pneumothorax where the patient's condition changes in seconds. But from the time the problem starts (not from the time you notice it) you only have a couple of hours until that hypoxic code. If it is 3 am and you are thinking the doctor will be here at 7 am—you don't have that kind of time. You need to move faster.

The fact that oxygen does not make it better is your first *big* sign that what you are dealing with is ARDS and not something else. If you ever put oxygen on a patient and do not see the PO_2 or O_2 sat respond to the increase in inspired oxygen, go directly to 100% oxygen. With ARDS, oxygen does not make it better. It is a life-threatening hypoxia that oxygen does not rectify.

The first clue that we might be looking at ARDS is that oxygen does not make it better. The second clue is the patient's breath sounds. They are unremarkable for such a severe hypoxia. They are *not* clear, but they do not give you a clue to the cause of the severe hypoxia. If you had a patient who was incredibly hypoxic when you put your stethoscope on his chest, you would expect to hear terrible things, like an absence of breath sounds, or unequal sounds signifying a pneumothorax or effusions, or nasty mucus rattling around. But the breath sounds are unremarkable. Not clear, but unremarkable for such an incredible hypoxia. You hear them all the way down both sides. They may be a little coarse or bronchial. Maybe a wheeze here or a rale there, but nothing that would account for the severity of the hypoxia. Let me tell you why.

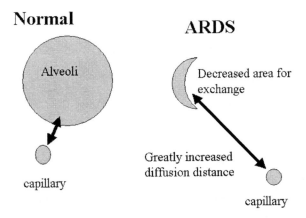

Just as in CHF, the patient going into ARDS will first swell up the interstitium between the alveolar wall and the capillary before dumping a lot of fluid and debris into the alveolus where it can be heard with a stethoscope. This swelling increases the distance the oxygen has to diffuse to make it into the capillary, and it compresses the size of the alveolar space where gas exchange takes place. The net result is a patient with a severe hypoxia, but with unremarkable breath sounds.

The blood gas showed a respiratory alkalosis. People with a respiratory alkalosis are frequently breathing too fast. The most common cause of hyperventilation is hypoxia, and being hypoxic will make you *very* anxious!

In the early stages of the disease we will see the patient blowing off CO_2 as he hyperventilates from the severe hypoxia. Because CO_2 exchanges across the alveolar membrane 20 times faster than oxygen does, the patient has destroyed a great deal of lung tissue before he begins to retain CO_2. Anytime a patient is retaining CO_2 there has been a tremendous loss of lung functioning and the end is near.

The heart rate on these patients goes up. Can you think of three things that could be driving the patient's heart rate up? Hypoxia will increase the heart rate as the heart speeds up the delivery system for oxygen to the tissues. Sympathetic stimulation causes the confused, restless, agitated, and combative response to hypoxia. Move into the patient's heart. When he got so incredibly hypoxic, his heart's contractility decreased. Stroke volume went down. To compensate for this loss in cardiac output, the heart rate goes up. Fluid lost through the capillary walls decreases return to the heart (preload) with a resultant loss of stroke volume, and again heart rate will rise. CO = HR × SV. These are things driving the patient's heart rate up.

And speaking of agitated, why is this patient so agitated? Yes, he's hypoxic. This is very easy to understand in a learning situation, but what if you are having a busy day? Mrs. Jones has just dc'd her IV again and has bled all over the bed, you have to call Dr. Intimidation and tell him how you accidentally pulled out his surgical patient's J-tube while changing his gown, and meanwhile, you have this patient down the hall saying unkind things about you and your mother.

This patient has a particularly nasty mouth, tattoos all over, and earrings in places you wouldn't dream of putting an earring. He is restless and combative. What could be wrong with this patient? Drug withdrawal, right? Maybe, but before you drag out the Haldol, please make sure he isn't hypoxic. The patients most likely to have their hypoxia missed are the ones with the psych or drug history. Always make sure your confused, restless, agitated, or combative patient is not hypoxic before proceeding.

The ARDS patient with the best chance of survival is the one that had his problem detected early. What does the patent going into ARDS look like? It is an acute onset of life threatening hypoxia that oxygen does not make better. Breath sounds are unremarkable for such an incredible hypoxia. The only way the patient is going to make it is if he can get into the unit, on a vent, before he has his hypoxic code.

Headaches

7

When the average person has a headache, chances are that it is an okay kind of headache. But, our patients aren't average people. They are the sick, infirm, and diseased; and if one of them says to us that she has a headache, chances are greater that it could be a malignant headache. Let's look at the differences between benign and malignant (or malevolent) headaches.

Malignant Headache

- First headache in patient over 35 years old
- No precipitating factor or starts with exercise and doesn't stop
- Awakens patient from sleep
- Thunderclap onset
- Dull, persistent pain
- Unilateral or focal pain accompanied by fever, change in LOC, papilledema, change in neuro signs, or meningeal signs
- No response to medication
- No pediatric history of motion sickness
- No family history of headache

Did you know that there are people who have never had a headache? Did you know there are whole families of people who have never had a headache in their lives? If someone is over 35 years old and has never had a headache in his entire life—and now has one—chances are it has a malevolent cause. One woman told me that no one in her family had headaches. Her mother had her first headache when she was 55 years old. It was the work-up for that headache that found her polycythemia. So if your patient has never had a headache and now has one, this is a clue that should not be ignored.

A headache that has no precipitating factor, or starts when you are exercising and doesn't stop when you stop exercising, is not usually benign in origin. Bad headaches that awaken you from sleep or have a thunderclap onset (sudden intense pain without gradual buildup), and dull, persistent pain that doesn't move around very much is a sign of a malevolent headache.

Unilateral or focal pain accompanied by fever, change in LOC, papilledema, change in neuro signs, or meningeal signs is a malevolent headache. If a patient tells a nurse she has a headache, very few of us stop and grab quick neuro signs, but we should. I know of a hospital that gave a family a whole bunch of money because a patient's headache did have a change in neuro signs, no nurse checked for it, and the diagnosis was missed. Our patients are sicker than ever before, so the chances that there have been changes in neuro signs is greater than ever before.

Headaches that do not respond to medication are not good headaches. A pediatric history of motion sickness is related to the development of migraines in later life. If you want to know if you had a history of motion sickness as a child, try to recall family car trips. Did you get nauseated? If you did, then you do, and you are at risk to develop migraines as you get older.

Benign Headache

- Patient less than 35 years old for first one
- Precipitating factors well known
- Previous similar headaches
- Pain disappears with sleep
- Gradual onset
- Pain describes as an ice pick, jab, or squeezing
- Multifocal and/or shifting sides
- No associated systemic or neurological findings except migraine aura

- Good response to medication
- Pediatric history of motion sickness (migraine)
- Positive family history

You and I have the good headaches. We've had them all our lives; we know exactly what causes them. We've had thousands of them. If we can get to sleep, our headaches usually go away (although migraine sufferers can wake up with their headaches intact). It has a gradual onset, and feels like the tops of our heads are blowing off. Medication *does* make it better, we barfed in the back seat of the car, and headaches are not unknown in our families. Those are the good ones.

Pain Patterns and Headaches

- Mild onset, worsening over 1 hr then abating—migraine and tension
- Moderate at onset present on awakening, abating—arterial hypertension, sinusitis
- Worst at onset Thunderclap HA—Subarachnoid hemorrhage (persistent), Cluster HA (abating)
- Pain awakening patient at night—Cluster headache
- Pain awakening patient in the morning—neoplasm, subarachnoid bleed
- New headache, worse over time—brain abscess, meningitis
- Chronic episodic headache—Migraine, cluster, tension, or sinus HA

Headaches that start out mild, get worse, and then get better are the good ones. Headaches that are there when you wake up in the morning, but get better as you are up running around can be arterial hypertension, but are more likely sinus in origin. Sinus headaches get better as you are up and about because they drain, and the pressure and pain goes away. People who suffer from sinus headaches know that laying down flat for a long time will bring them on; being in air conditioning will do it; and having oxygen blown up your nose will occlude your sinuses in nothing flat. (And what do we do in hospitals? We bring people into air-conditioned rooms, lay them down flat, and blow oxygen up their noses!)

You don't want to throw pain medication at someone's sinus headache, you'll just nauseate them. You want to open up their sinuses, and the pain will go away. You need to know if this patient's headache is a sinus headache. But how do you find out? Ask the patient to point to the center of the headache with one finger. If the patient points to an area including the eyes and forehead, it is probably a sinus headache. If he points to anywhere else, it is most likely not a sinus headache.

Headaches that are worse at onset or have a thunder clap onset—meaning there was no gradual lead up to the pain; it was all suddenly there in full force—can be subarachnoid bleeds or cluster headaches. If you have a cerebral aneurysm ready to go, all you need to do is cough, sneeze, or turn your head sharply and you can blow it wide open. I haven't turned my head sharply since I read that.

Cluster headaches are more frequently seen in men than women and are characterized by severe headaches that are episodic in nature. That is, there are periods of headaches, and periods of being headache-free. Clusters usually last 2 weeks to 3 months and are separated by at least 2-week intervals of calm. They tend to occur at the same time of the day, can wake you from a deep sleep, and can be more painful than migraines. The pain is unilateral, centered behind one eye, and is often accompanied by nausea and vomiting.

A new headache that gets worse over time requires a physician. If you have tension headaches, they all feel the same. Your sinus headaches all feel the same, as do your migraine headaches. A new type of headache is a medical emergency. Our patients usually don't differentiate between types of headaches. You have to ask the questions. *"Is this your usual and accustomed headache?" "Is it in the usual strength and duration?"* You must ask because our patients are sicker than ever and the chances that you have a malignant cause for the headache is greater.

The headache you get from increased intercranial pressure is like no headache you have ever felt before. It has been described as more global, more intense, and just plain old different from any other headache. People who have had increased intercranial pressure know what I mean. It is a totally different kind of headache.

Pain Characteristic vs. Cause

- Ocular lesion—Orbital or frontal worsening after eye use
- Vascular disorder—Throbs in time with the pulse and follows blood vessel

- Neurologic lesion (herpes zoster)—Pain follows nerve
- Deep, aching, relatively localized—Inflammation
- Localized to site of injury—Post traumatic reaction
- Ear pain with HA—Ear lesion
- Oral pain with HA—Oral lesion

Pain characteristics vary by cause of the headache also. Headaches that are suborbital or frontal and that worsen after eye use can be problems within the eye itself. Lesions of the nerves themselves, such as herpes zoster, can cause the pain of the headache to follow the affected nerve. The headache from vascular disorders can throb in time with the pulse and follow a blood vessel. These headaches will feel different from the patient's usual and accustomed headaches. Inflammation, getting hit on your head, and lesions in the ear and mouth can also cause headaches. These headaches will also feel different from the patient's usual and accustomed headaches.

Sign/Symptom vs. Cause

- Abnormal vision preceding HA—Migraine aura
- Abnormal vision after onset of HA—Occipital vascular malformation, other eye problem
- Horizontal double vision on near focusing, lid droop—Media rectus paresis (possible posterior communicating artery)
- Horizontal double vision on far focusing—Lateral rectus paresis (possible increased ICP)
- Horner's syndrome—Lesion of the sympathetic nervous system causing drooping eye lid, permanent constriction of the pupil, and you don't sweat on that side of your face. Transient—Cluster HA; Persistent—Carotid artery dissection
- Nausea and vomiting—Too much pain medication, increased ICP, migraine, meningitis, toxicity
- Fever—Infectious or toxic origin
- Change in LOC, focal neurological deficit—Malignant cause, especially neoplasm or subarachnoid bleed
- Papilledema—Increased ICP
- Neck and back pain—Meningitis, subarachnoid bleed

If you have abnormal vision before the headache starts, don't worry about it. It is probably migraine aura. If the abnormal vision starts up *after* the headache begins, it could have a more sinister cause. It could be caused by an occipital vascular malformation or some other eye problem. It might be a problem with the posterior communicating artery, or it could be increased intercranial pressure.

Horner's syndrome occurs from a lesion of the sympathetic nervous system, causing a drooping eye lid, permanent constriction of the pupil, and inability to sweat on that side of the face. It can occur with cluster headaches and be transient. If it is persistent, it can be a sign of carotid artery dissection.

Nausea and vomiting with a headache can be a sign of increased intercranial pressure, migraine, meningitis, or toxicity, but a more common cause is too much medication for the headache on an empty stomach. Always ask the patient what he has taken for his headache. Sometimes he will say, *"Well, I took about 8 aspirin before I took some of that ibuprofen stuff. Then my wife had some Tylenol with codeine left over from her surgery and I had two of them and a couple of Demerol tablets my cousin gave me yesterday."* No wonder the guy is nauseated! Before assuming increased intercranial pressure, always ask patients what they took for the headache.

If there is a fever with a headache, it can have an infectious or toxic origin. Remember, you activate the response to injury to clean up debris and chemicals. If the headache is accompanied by a change in LOC, papilledema, or focal neurological deficit, absolutely nothing good can be causing it. You need a doctor. Neck and back pain can be meningitis, it can also be a subarachnoid bleed.

Causes of increased intercranial pressure

- Neoplasm or tumor
- Hydrocephalus
- Pseudo tumor cerebri
- Venous stasis occlusion
- Vascular disorder
- Pressure from benign exertion

Your head is a fixed space. There is room for a certain amount of blood, gray matter, and cerebral spinal fluid. If either of those three things becomes greater in volume than it should be, or if the circumference of the head becomes smaller, you get an increase in intercranial pressure. The cause of the increase in pressure can be easily seen for all the above conditions *except* pseudo tumor cerebri. This is an idiopathic (meaning we don't know the reason it happens) intra-cranial hypertension caused because the patient doesn't reabsorb his spinal fluid the way he should. It causes a headache with a visual defect.

Temporal Arteritis

- Continuous throbbing frontal HA
- Repetitive needle like pains
- Scalp tenderness
- Jaw claudication
- Temporal artery tenderness
- Diminished temporal pulses
- Visual disturbance
- Fever & elevated sed rate

Temporal arteritis is a very nasty headache. It is continuous and constant. If you give the patient narcotics, it will knock him out, and when he awakens, the headache is still right there with all its intensity. This headache is caused by an inflammation of the temporal artery. If you are looking for it in the patient, you might be able to see a low grade fever and elevated sed rate. Definitive diagnosis is made with a temporal artery biopsy, which is not something you rush out and do to everyone with a bad headache. Because it is inflammatory, Prednisone is the drug of choice, not something you rush out an do to everyone with a bad headache, either. Some people get their diagnosis made when they lose the vision in one of their eyes.

Primary and Secondary Headaches

Primary Headaches
- Migraine
- Cluster
- Muscle contraction
- Miscellaneous not associated with a structural lesion

Secondary Headaches
- Head trauma
- Vascular disorders
- Nonvascular inter-cranial disorder
- Substance use or withdrawal
- Non-cephalic infection
- Metabolic disorder
- Disorder of cranium, facial or cranial structure
- Neuralgia, nerve trunk pain

Headaches can have a primary cause such as migraine, muscle contraction, or structural lesions. In these events, the headache is a direct reflection of the event. Some headaches, however, are secondary to other things. For example, getting hit on the head can cause a headache. Vascular disorders and substance use or withdrawal (most notably caffeine) can cause headaches. Infections in places other than your head (the non-healing ulcer on your foot) via toxins can cause a headache. Metabolic disorders such as having your lytes, BUN and Cr, or a poorly functioning liver can cause headaches. Anything that keeps your spinal fluid from draining as it should, disorders of the cranium, facial or cranial structure, and neuralgia and nerve trunk pain can also cause headaches.

Headaches can have many causes, and be benign or malignant in nature. Because our patients frequently do not differentiate one headache from another, we must always remember to ask, *"Is this your usual and accustomed headache? Is it different in any way?"* Remember to grab quick neuro signs to prove there hasn't been a change. If the answer to either of these questions indicates a different or more intense headache than usual, or there has been a change in LOC or neuro signs, call the doctor.

The Look Test

8

I f someone says to you that your patient doesn't look right, what does that mean? Maybe you just "feel" something isn't quite as it should be. What is this thing called nurse's intuition? Nurses knew they had intuition, but they didn't know how to describe it until two nurses, Benner and Tanner, did a study. They discovered that a nurse's "intuition" was rapid critical thinking based on his or her past experience. Every time you had ever seen a patient look that way or act that way, nothing good had ever come of it!

When we talk about how a patient *looks*, what things are we discussing? The following has been compiled with the help of many nurses, with many years of experience. These nurses were asked for clues they had noticed over the years that indicate a patient isn't doing very well. The result is *The Look Test*.

The Look Test

- Color
- Effort—Fatigability
- Skin—Diaphoresis
- Mentation
- Increased HR, increased RR
- Frightened ("Don't leave me")

One of the first things you notice about patients is their color. Skin color is a factor of pigmentation and oxygenation and perfusion in the capillaries. People are *not* supposed to change color. They are to stay the color God gave them, and if they start changing color it is a very bad sign. I once watched a patient in the ER turn a rainbow of colors never realizing that the change in color was heralding his imminent cardiac arrest. If your patient changes color, it is a sign of bad things— like a failure to oxygenate and perfuse at the same time, leading to a lethal dysrhythmia.

We didn't used to care so much if a patient was breathing really fast to keep his O_2 sat at 95%. We were just happy he had a sat of 95%. Well, now we care a great deal about the effort the patient is putting out to keep his numbers where they are because we recognize fatigability to be a real crisis generator. How hard is the patient working to keep those numbers up? How long do you think he will be able to keep going?

We now recognize diaphoresis to be a sign of maximal sympathetic stimulation, and as such, a sign of impending doom. We also look for subtle changes in mentation. Or maybe the heart rate and respiratory rate have increased, but there isn't any other change. An increase in heart rate and respiratory rate are your first two compensatory mechanisms. When they fail, that's when you get abnormal clinical signs.

We have all experienced the patient who appears frightened and says, *"Don't leave me!"* You are very aware of how things are going in your body at all times. You know your own "normal." You take this information and put it into your subconscious because you have a life to live, and you can't deal with this information on a minute-to-minute basis.

This information on your body's functioning stays in your subconscious until something goes wrong. When that happens, it comes immediately to the forefront of your consciousness and gives you a sympathetic stimulation. This is what causes these patients' frightened, wide-eyed, and agitated appearance. Anyone who says to you, *"Don't leave me!"* is trying to tell you they have had that sympathetic stimulation. They probably can't tell you what is wrong, just that something is definitely *not right*. They are trying to warn you that they are receiving a subclinical sign of their impending doom.

Pay attention to people who tell you they aren't going to make it through this event. I know a surgeon who won't operate if a patient tells him she doesn't feel like she is going to make it. He's had too many people die after telling him that. You are much more attuned to your body that you think you are. Some people seem know when they are going to die. Nurses see it over and over again. *Pay attention.*

- Eyes
- Smell
- Nurse just senses something's not right

People's eyes sparkle. The sparkle-o-meter runs from +4 to dull and glazed over. On any given day, you and I sparkle at about a +3. You make it to +4 if you are happy or delighted. If you are getting sick, your eyes don't sparkle quite as much as they used to. You may have noticed that in your children. Before they give you concrete signs that, indeed, they are headed into another ear infection, strep throat, or whatever, their eyes don't sparkle like they usually do.

Did you know that there are people who can smell a patient getting ready to code? *What?! Smell a patient getting ready to code?* We have animals that can be trained to detect lots of things. We have bomb sniffing, cadaver, and rescue dogs. There are animals that have been trained to sense when their owners are getting ready to have seizures. The animal gives a signal and the owner lies down so he doesn't fall down and hurt himself. Animals have been trained to sense when a diabetic's blood sugar is dropping off precipitously. They give a signal and the owner checks his blood sugar.

"But," you say, "*those are animals.*" But we are animals too. Who says we can't smell and sense a lot of what other animals do. Just like dogs and other animals, some humans smell and sense better than other humans. I, personally, can't smell acetone breath. Meanwhile, other people are gagging in the hallway.

Healthcare workers in third world countries are taught to smell the differences in diseases and the differences in infections. We smell it too, but in America we spend most of our time trying to cover up smells. We had the privilege of ignoring smells because we had lab tests to tell us what was going on with our patients. It was never important to learn what smell might indicate, but over time we have learned associations. Can you smell cancer on a patient? C diff? Pseudomonas? Strep throat?

If I ask people who say they can smell a patient getting ready to code what it smells like, overwhelmingly I get the same answer. The first response is, *"Well . . . ummm . . . it's hard to describe."* Apparently it is a very distinctive, very unpleasant smell, like no other. If you inquire further, the nurse will describe it as a very unpleasant, sweet, musty smell. Like socks that have been in a gym bag at school for a year. One nurse said it reminds her of rancid body odor, but that it is a distinctive odor unto itself. Another said it smelled earthy, like mushrooms.

Just like animals vary in their ability to smell, so do humans. Some nurses claim to smell patients with electrolyte imbalances or fluid overload. Every disease has its own particular smell, but we were never taught what we were smelling. Animals may sense more than we do, but I think we just don't pay enough attention to what we sense. We get "feelings" about situations, but we ignore the information because we are looking for things we can talk to the doctor about—concrete signs, not "feelings." Those feelings are a large part of nurse's intuition. Pay attention to them. If you feel uneasy, respect that. It is valuable data.

- Family
- Voice
- Change in activity level
- Preoccupied
- Picking

Nursing school is full of family—the support of family, the joy and wonder of family, and all we want is for them to go home. *"He's feeling better now. Why don't you go home? There's nothing more you can do for him. Why don't you go home?"* All this is said with the best of intentions, but when the family leaves so does the history of that patient and that patient's support group. Unconscious people may be aware of people around them. Try your best to include the family. I know it increases the stress involved in taking care of the patient, but it is the family who knows what this person is supposed to walk like, talk like, and provides the emotional support for the patient. There are exceptions, of course, where the family is a negative factor, but not that often.

The trouble with family is that we tend to think of them as ignorant and in the way. Have you ever noticed that when you are the nurse standing at the bedside, you're pretty smart. But, as soon as you sit down at your mother's bedside you become brain dead? The health care staff are the keepers of the knowledge, and the family are the lucky recipients of our collective wisdom if they obey the rules and are lucky. Over the years we have gotten much, much better at including family at the bedside. We still have a way to go in learning to listen to them when they tell us Uncle George isn't looking or behaving in his normal way. Listen to the family! They know these people; we don't.

You can tell a great deal about people from their voices. You can tell oxygenation and perfusion from the strength of the voice and clarity of ideas. You can also tell tidal volume from someone's voice. It has to do with the number of words you can string together in a sentence. If you can string a bunch of them together, you have good volume. If you start making very short sentences or taking a breath every few words, your tidal volume and/or oxygenation is decreasing. You can also hear sympathetic stimulation as fear in the patient's voice if you are listening for it.

Any patient who has had a sudden change in activity level is talking to you. That can be the antsy patient who is suddenly calm, or the calm patient who is suddenly antsy. The patient who was preoccupied as you were walking around his room—that's not normal. He should be paying close attention to you. He's not oxygenating and perfusing quite as well as he was before. Nor is the patient who is picking at everything.

- The numbers don't add up
- Having "a better day"
- Visits from the dead
- Sees a religious figure
- Hungry at an odd time

Vital signs fit together in groups. Good, bad, or ugly, they fit into their assigned group. But, what if you get a number that doesn't fit? You have a patient who is blue, respiratory rate and heart rate are both up, but the O_2 sat is 98%. What do you do? Retake your numbers, look for variables, and if things are still not adding up, ask for what I like to call a *nursing consult*. A nursing consult is where you turn to the nurse next to you and say, *"What do you think?"* Some of us seem to think that we can't ask for help because it will show our lack of knowledge and decrease our status. The highest form of nursing is one practiced with lots of nursing consults. The lowest form of nursing is the lone ranger approach.

When you look at numbers, always ask yourself, *"Who generated this number?"* Nurse's aides frequently generate numbers that the nurse acts upon. If a number is not fitting into its grouping—go take it yourself. If you send the nurse's aide back to retake it, she might simply make the same mistake again.

Some nurse's aides have received a very poor education in how to take a pulse oximetry reading. You'll see them go into the patient's room, slip the probe onto the finger, and turn the machine on. They take the very first number that pops up—particularly if it is a good number—whip the probe off the finger, and they are out the door. As you well know, if the patient's apical heart rate is not correlated to the heart rate on the machine, or if you have a very brisk pleth, the number is garbage.

It is also considered cheating to hyperventilate the patient into a good number. *"Bertha take a breath! That's good. Do it again. Okay, deeper, deeper. One more time. That's good!"* And you whip the probe off the finger, and out the door you go while Bertha once again hypoventilates. You want the number to reflect where the patient is, not where you occasionally stimulate them to be.

Watch the patient who is suddenly having a better day. You could be looking at the last cathecolamine surge where the body takes everything it has left and summons up one last effort to stay alive. This is the patient who has been sick as a dog, and then one morning he sits up, eats with a good appetite, has a lovely chat with relatives, and dies the next day. Nurses see this over and over again.

Visits from the dead can be a very bad sign. The patient's husband has been dead for six years. Now he is sitting on the end of the bed talking to her. This is a very bad sign. He has probably come to take her with him down the tunnel. Seeing a religious figure is also bad. If the patient is Christian and looks up and starts talking to Jesus or to angels, the situation is deteriorating.

Pay attention to the patient who is hungry at an odd time. A Type II diabetic on oral medications has been admitted to the hospital to have cardiac meds started up. It is 1 o'clock in the afternoon. He calls his nurse and says, *"I'm hungry. Can I have something to eat?"* The nurse says, *"Why are you hungry? You just had lunch and you ate everything. I know because I picked up your tray."* To which the patient replied, *"I don't know. I'm just hungry. Okay?"*

What this nurse knew was that when a diabetic's blood sugar is dropping, there is a zone at which, no matter when this patient last put food in his mouth, he becomes hungry. Knowing this, she checked the patient's blood sugar and it was 45. This zone of hunger has a bottom to it. If a diabetic ever asks for something to eat and you can't get it to him right away, and you go back later and the diabetic claims to no longer be hungry, check his blood sugar. That zone of hunger has a bottom to it, and if the patient doesn't eat he can fall right out of the hunger zone into the "I'm in big trouble" zone while still appearing to be just fine, because all he is doing is lying in bed. We tend to think that if the patient is talking to us the sugar can't be too bad. What is the lowest blood sugar you have had on a patient who is talking to you? Forty? Thirty? Twenty!

- Ear and nose cartilage relaxes
- Loss of discomfort
- Heavenward gaze in unconscious patient
- Blue knees
- The patient who is afraid of going to bed

Some nurses have noticed that before a patient dies the ear and nose cartilage relaxes. Your ears are firm and stick out from the sides of your head. Because of this, they are ideal for supporting nasal cannula. Right before death, because of oxygenation and perfusion—and the lack thereof—the cartilage becomes soft. Some nurses say the ears lay back against the head. Others say they curl up from the bottom or curl down from the tops, but you notice it happening when you can't keep the cannula on the patient's ears any more and have to start taping it to the cheeks.

Then there is the patient that you have to medicate for pain every time it's possible. You can never get this patient comfortable. If the time comes for his medication and he doesn't need it any more, the situation could be deteriorating.

When you have an unconscious patient, every few hours you do neuro checks where you look at the patient's pupils. You open the eyes to shine your light into the pupils and the eyes are right there looking back at you. The next time you come along and raise the eyelids you see that the eyes have rolled back in the patient's head. That is the heavenward gaze in the unconscious patient, indicating that things have deteriorated.

Mottling anywhere in the body is a bad idea, and one of the first places patients mottle is the kneecaps. Blue knees are a bad sign. Then there are the patients who won't go to bed. It is as if they feel that if they get into bed, lay down, and go to sleep ,they are going to die. Now that's silly, isn't it? People don't know when they are going to die, do they? Many nurses will say, *"Yes, they do."* Some patients seem to have a premonition of their deaths and contact family members for a last chat before they pass on unexpectedly.

- Can't get O_2 Sat any more
- Can't hold body temperature
- Soles of feet in a code
- Craving ice
- Last face

The pulse oximetry that had been working just fine no longer seems able to find the patient's pulse, and it keeps alarming. Some nurses have been known to turn off the alarms thinking it was a malfunctioning machine. But what's happening is that perfusion is decreasing into that extremity. *Check the patient!*

The patient who can't hold his body temperature up is another sign of impending doom.

A nurse told me that she could tell if a patient was going to make it through a code based on the color of the soles of his feet. If the feet were gray he wasn't going to make it, and if the feet *weren't* gray he probably *was* going to make it. I'm sure it has to do with the degree of oxygenation and circulatory shutdown.

What is the patient who craves ice trying to tell you? She could be anemic. Anemics are well known to crave ice. This is called ice pica. It isn't the contents of the ice—you could get that by drinking the water. It has something to do with the crunch. When you are anemic, you crave ice. When you're not, you don't.

Another group that craves ice are patients whose tanks are empty. If all the nurse will give them is ice chips, they will take gallons of ice and try to fill their tanks back up. This is why some post-op, hemorrhaging, or trauma patients can crave ice.

- Black dog

We have done very little study of end of life experiences. If the patient sees something we don't see, we assume they are confused and hallucinating. But, what if many patients see the *same* hallucination? I have been told of numerous incidences where nurses were told by patients that they saw a black dog in their rooms before they died. One nurse learned of the black dog when her patient said, *"I didn't know you allowed pets in the ICU."* The nurse asked, *"What pet?"* The patient replied, *"That black dog over in the corner."*

The very interesting thing about the black dog is that the patients frequently reported seeing the same black dog. It is the size of a German shepherd or a lab with medium length black hair. It has been reported to be in the corner, under the bed, on the bed, or outside a window looking in at the patient. Its presence is usually benign, and the patients don't mind it being there. One patient slept with her arm around the dog. Another one reported that the dog came running up to him, put its head on his lap, and looked up at him adoringly.

All these patients died. Not every dying patient sees the black dog, but some do. What is the significance of the black dog? It appears in religious myths from all around the world, and it always has to do with the death experience. We have done very little study of end of life experiences, and here is some nursing research just waiting to happen.

Functions of
the Kidneys

9

Functions of the Kidneys

- Eliminate metabolic waste
    urea
    creatinine
    uric acid
- Regulate extracellular volume
- Osmolality of body fluids
- Electrolyte balance
- Acid-base balance
- Secrete hormones
    renin
    erythropoietin
    prostaglandins
- Gluconeogenesis—glucose from amino acids

Your kidneys are responsible for excreting the waste products of our metabolic functioning. They regulate volume and osmolality of the body's fluids, they balance electrolyes and pH, and secrete hormones.

Now, I want you to believe that your kidneys regulate your blood pressure and your hematocrit. This would make no sense at all if you had discrete organ systems that functioned independently of each other. But you don't. You have one set of completely interrelated organs. So of course the kidneys can regulate your blood pressure and your hematocrit if they want to.

The kidneys are also capable of gluconeogenesis—making new sugar from amino acids. In a time of crisis, like shock, they can scrape together the components of ATP and try to keep themselves alive. This is how important they are to the body.

BUN	Creatinine	Diagnosis
⬆	Normal or slightly ↑	Volume depletion or poor perfusion
⬆	Normal or slightly ↑	Protein catabolism
⬆	⬆	Kidney disease

THE PATIENT WITH A HIGH BUN

When you look at someone's kidney function, you look at the BUN and Creatinine (Cr). If both the BUN and Cr are up, you have someone with renal dysfunction. But there are two other things that make the BUN go up, but not the Cr. The first one, you see all the time: volume depletion. An elderly lady comes in dehydrated, and her BUN is high. You rehydrate her, and in the next day or so her BUN falls to normal. This is a concentration issue.

The other group with a high BUN but without renal failure are patients who have a lot of protein to metabolize. Earlier we said that an end product of protein metabolism was BUN. Patients with crushing injuries have a lot of myoglobin to metabolize and excrete, as do burn and trauma patients. Patients with red blood cells outside of the blood vessels but still within their body—hematomas, GI bleeds, trauma, etc.—have large amounts of protein to be metabolized. With these patients you expect to see the BUN go up, but not the Cr. When both are up you have kidney problems.

IS HE WET OR IS HE DRY?

Is he wet or is he dry? How do you tell? The answer to this question drove Drs. William Ganz and Jeremy Swan to invent their famous catheter in the 1970s. When the first Swan-Ganz catheters came out, they came with a questionnaire asking doctors to guess whether they thought their patients were wet or dry. Then, they were to put the catheter in and tell the researchers what numbers they got. The results showed that 50% of the time the doctors guessed wrong. But why can't you tell?

Fluid Depletion
- tachycardia
- variable BP
- ↓ urine output
- dry mucus membranes
- ↑ thirst

Fluid Overload
- tachycardia
- variable BP
- ↓ urine output
- rales
- edema
- Metabolic disorder
- hypoxia, dyspnea
- JVD

The problem is the signs and symptoms. The first three are identical for both groups. When a patient is over-loaded *and* when a patient is under-loaded, the heart rate goes up because stroke volume falls off, so that is not an indicator. Because of vasoconstriction, blood pressure is not a good indicator. Both groups also stop urinating. So how do you know?

You can rely on thirst as an indicator of volume depletion *only* if you have a patient with an intact thirst mechanism and the ability to ask for a glass of water. You don't always get that. If you live long enough, everything in your body is going to fail you, including your thirst mechanism. No one has to tell a young person to get a drink. They have brisk thirst mechanisms. But as you get older it looses its vigor. This is why elderly people so often end up in the hospital with dehydration. They don't know to take a drink. If you work with these people, you are constantly offering them something to drink and they are constantly saying, *"No thank you. I'm not thirsty."* You must constantly encourage them to drink.

But you can tell if a patient is over-hydrated can't you, because they have rales, edema, shortness of breath, and hypoxia, right? But rales, edema, shortness of breath, and hypoxia can each be caused by lots of things, and they are not characteristic only to fluid overload.

JUGULAR VENOUS DISTENTION

The only useful sign of over-hydration is jugular venous distention (JVD). In the absence of right heart failure it is JVD that tells you the patient is fluid over-loaded. You can call the doctor and describe low sats, rapid heart rates, swollen ankles, and wet lungs, but all of those signs can have multiple causes. The things that can cause positive JVD are constrictive pericarditis, inferior vena cava obstruction, severe tricuspid regurgitation, cardiac tamponade, massive pulmonary embolus, superior vena cava syndrome, right heart failure, and fluid overload. The ones you are most likely to run into are right heart failure and fluid overload. In the absence of right heart failure, the most likely cause of positive JVD is fluid overload.

Most nurses don't know how to measure JVD, so let me explain.

What you are looking for is the external jugular vein that runs up the side of the neck. You have the patient at a 30–45 degree elevation (depending on which author you read) resting in bed. Then you look to see if you can *see* the vein. Do not palpate. If you have a patient with a fat neck, you may need to turn the head or pull the skin. If you have an extremely thin patient, you may always see their veins. They are little anatomy lessons just laying there. But, for the average patient this method will work just fine.

So we have the patient in bed, the head of the bed raised 45 degrees, and we look to see if the vein can be seen. If you can see it, how many finger widths does it take to cover it up? JVD is measured in +1, +2, +3, or +4. A JVD of +1 means it takes the width of one finger placed horizontally to cover the vein; +3 means it takes three finger widths, etc. The zero point is the top of the patient's clavicle. Find the top of the clavicle, look for the vein, see how many fingers it takes to cover it up, put a + sign in front of how many fingers it takes, and there is your measurement.

Zero to +1 is normal. You cannot see fluid deficit because the vein falls down into the chest and most of us can't see into the chest, so JVD is good for fluid overload only. You will see doctors check JVD on patients sitting up in chairs. If you have +JVD sitting up, you definitely have +JVD in bed at a 45 degree angle. Patients with fluid overload are frequently in respiratory distress, and sitting up lowers the amount of blood returning into the heart (preload), thereby decreasing CHF symptoms. Asking the patient to get into bed, put his feet on the bed, and his head down to a 45 degree angle can precipitate a respiratory and / or cardiac crisis. If they don't have +JVD sitting up, it doesn't mean they won't have it at a 45 degree angle in bed. One does not preclude the other in this case.

The Effects of Surgical Trauma

10

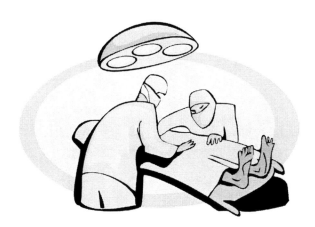

The Body's Regulatory Systems

- Autoregulation GFR
- RAAS
- Aldosterone
- Antidiuretic hormone
- Baroreceptors
- Volume receptors
- Atrial natriuretic factor
- Osmoreceptors

The name of the game is homeostasis, and the body has all kinds of regulatory systems designed to keep you in homeostasis. The first item on the list above is something called autoregulation within the capillary beds. Your capillaries are one cell thick at their smallest. This is a very fragile system. If every time your blood pressure increased, that increase in pressure had been transmitted into those capillaries, you would have blown them all apart by now. When you go to sleep your blood pressure drops and flow in the capillaries slows. But when blood slows down, it clots. It is *supposed* to, but it can make getting out of bed in the morning very difficult!

Dorland's Medical Dictionary defines autoregulation as:

1. The process occurring when some mechanism within a biological system detects and adjusts for changes within the system; exercised by negative feedback.

2. In circulatory physiology, the intrinsic tendency of an organ or tissue to maintain constant blood flow despite changes in arterial pressure, or the adjustment of blood flow through an organ in order to provide for its metabolic needs.

Capillary Bed

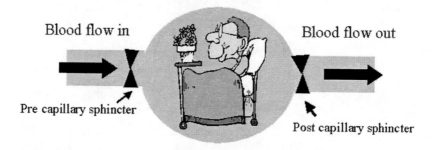

Blood flow in   Blood flow out

Pre capillary sphincter   Post capillary sphincter

PRE- AND POST-CAPILLARY SPHINCTERS

We have pre- and post-capillary sphincters that respond to various chemicals and metabolic events to open and close the sphincters and regulate blood flow through the capillaries.

By opening and closing the sphincters, it is possible to protect the delicate capillary bed from systolic pressures up to 180 mmHg and all the way down to a systolic pressure of 80 mmHg. The same degree of flow can be maintained throughout this continuum. Here's how it works. If the arterial pressure is increasing, you constrict the pre-capillary sphincter to reduce the pressure into the capillary bed while at the same time you open the post-capillary sphincter to let the pressure out the other side. Physiologists think this process is driven not only by stretch receptors but also by the metabolic need of the tissues fed by this capillary.

The system works in the reverse also. If the arterial pressure is dropping, the pre-capillary sphincter opens while the post-capillary one closes. This increases the pressure within the capillary bed. It ca also cause capillary sludging where flow slows in the affected capillaries and the clotting cascade is activated. This is a wonderful way to get disseminated intravascular coagulaopathy (DIC). It is important to keep the patient's pressure up to prevent DIC.

The autoregulation mentioned in the list says "GFR." GFR refers to the glomeral filtration rate in the kidney. Autoregulation protects the delicate nephron and its capillary from damage from systolic pressures up to 180 mmHg and all the way down to a systolic pressure of 80 mmHg.

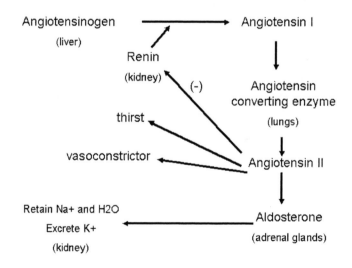

The renin angiotensin aldosterone system (RAAS) is simply a marvel. The kidneys don't know that they aren't part of the cardiovascular system. When blood flows into the kidney, it measures the pressure with something called the justaglomeral apparatus. If the pressure is down, it causes the kidney to secrete renin, which goes out into the circulatory system looking for the angiotensinogen that was placed there by the liver. The two combine and turn themselves into angiotensin I which goes rushing off to the lungs looking for the angiotensin converting enzyme, finds it, and turns itself in angiotensin II.

Angiotensin II has multiple effects in the body, but there are two effects in particular that we are interested in: 1) it goes off to the brain, causes the release of ACTH, which goes to the adrenal gland causing the secretion of aldosterone, which goes to the kidney causing the renal tubule to retain sodium and water, and 2) it is a very potent vasoconstrictor.

We just whipped our way through seven organ systems regulating your blood pressure. You do not have multiple sets of independent organ systems, you have *one set* of interrelated organs.

Another regulatory mechanism is the antidiuretic hormone (ADH). It is activated when there appears to be a need to retain water within the body, as with cases of stress, increased sodium levels, or hypotension. The stress response itself can cause the secretion of aldosterone and the retention of sodium and water by the kidneys. This is designed to increase blood volume at a time of stress, which would increase transport capacity and reserve.

There are little pressure plates called baroreceptors through out the body. There is a concentration of them in the arch of the aorta. They talk to the autonomic nervous system via sympathetic and parasympathetic nerve fibers. Homeostasis wants a nice even blood pressure—no spikes, no troughs. As the blood leaves the left ventricle and goes out into the aorta, the baroreceptors measure the blood pressure. If the pressure is going up, the body decreases the heart rate and vasodilates a little bit. If the pressure is going down, it increases the heart rate and vasoconstricts the blood vessels a bit. In this way you keep a nice even blood pressure. If the vascular volume is also dropping, it causes the secretion of ADH which in turn causes the kidneys to retain water and increases blood pressure.

There are volume and stretch receptors in the atria of the heart. When the atria are stretched by volume overload, these receptors cause the atria to secrete atrial natriuretic factor. The released peptide acts on the renal tubule, causing an excretion of sodium and water.

When the volume load goes down, the receptors return to normal. And of course, there are the ever-popular osmoreceptors that are tied directly into the thirst mechanism. These are the major regulatory systems that we know about today. Tomorrow, I'm sure we will know of more.

What are the effects of surgical trauma on the body's regulatory systems? Surgery is indeed trauma. It is *scheduled* trauma, but the effect is the same.

Surgery's Effect on the Regulatory Mechanisms

- General anesthesia
- Narcotics and fentanyl—vasodilators
- Succinylcholine—increase K+ levels
- halothane, sedatives and muscle relaxants—decrease myocardial contractility
- compensatory mechanisms a minimum of 24 hours (the longer the surgery the longer the effect)
- Blood and fluid loss → RAAS
- Third space fluid shifts
- Mechanical ventilation
- Hypothermia

If a patient gets a general anesthesia with surgery and receives narcotics and/or Fentanyl, these vasodilators can cause pressure and volume problems. The succinylcholine given to paralyze the patient so the ET tube can be inserted increases potassium levels. Anesthetic gasses such as halothane, sedatives, and muscle relaxants decrease myocardial contractility. The regulatory mechanisms are blunted for a minimum of 24 hours (the longer the surgery the longer the effect). Also, the more co-morbid factors going into the surgery and the more complications post-op, the longer the blunt.

When patients bleed from surgery they will set off the renin angiotensin aldosterone system, causing them to retain fluid and increase blood pressure. This is achieved by retaining sodium and water in the kidneys and by vasoconstriction of the blood vessels. If the patient retains sodium and water, it makes the preload in the heart go up—a bad idea in a patient with heart failure. Vasoconstriction makes the afterload of the heart go up—also a bad idea in a heart failure patient. Both of these normal compensatory mechanisms increase the work load of the heart.

Now, if you are a sweet young thing having surgery, this doesn't matter. Young, healthy people have lots of reserve. Unfortunately, there are many more tired, old people with bad hearts and lungs than there are healthy, young people in our hospitals and extended care facilities. The acknowledgement of these problems are why sick, elderly people don't get as much general anesthesia as they used to.

Because of increased capillary permeability from inflammation (the response to injury), patients move fluid into the tissues, which can leave the patient vascularly dry. Being on a ventilator can increase volumes within the chest, activating baro and volume receptors and stimulating the RAAS and ADH secretion, leading to an increase of sodium and water. You can get Syndrome of Inappropriate Antidiuretic Hormone (SIADH) simply by being placed on a ventilator.

The hypothermia you come out of the OR with decreases your metabolic needs, but it also decreases myocardial contractility, drops the heart rate, causes peripheral vasoconstriction (raising the work load of the heart), impairs insulin release, and stimulates the RAAS. This can cause hypertension, hyperglycemia, decreased cardiac output, and fluid and electrolyte imbalance. Not your favorite things to have happen to your elderly and/or frail patient.

THE EFFECTS OF SURGICAL TRAUMA
(SCHEDULED TRAUMA VS. UNSCHEDULED TRAUMA)

12 to 48 hrs post insult
• vascular depletion
• dry mucus membranes
• edema
• weight gain
• ↑ serum glucose
• ↓ K +
• cool pale skin
• irregular HR

When the surgeon takes the knife and makes an incision into the skin, it is an injury. It's no different than if you accidentally cut yourself. You set off the response to injury: the capillaries vasodilate, the slit pores open up, and out goes the fluid. Because of this you are now volume depleted. This is why patients receive so much fluid in surgery and recovery. They are trying to fill the patient's tank back up. Unfortunately, you can overfill the tank, throwing the patient into CHF. It is a delicate balance sometimes.

Because the slit pores opened up and the fluid poured out, your patient is edematous. Edema is no indicator of fluid overload in the post-op patient. They are *all* edematous because of the response to injury. This is also why patients gain weight post-op. Each liter of fluid weighs 2.2 pounds.

Because of the stress response and your glucocorticoids, your serum glucose is abnormal. Because of the stress response and your minerocorticoids, your electrolytes are abnormal. These are two of the four things (normal pH, balanced electrolytes, oxygen and glucose inside the cell being used to make ATP) that can lead to a lethal dysrhythmia. This a delicate situation requiring an observant nurse.

---

24 to 72 hours post-insult (reabsorption/diuresis phase)

- decreased capillary permeability
- decreased third spacing
- increased vascular volume
- Na+ excess
- K+ depletion

The patient has survived the immediate post-op period and she is going home tomorrow. You are looking at making out assignments for the night shift. Can you give her to the weakest nurse on the floor? Yes, you do. You have to give them someone; you can't take care of the whole floor. Besides, she is mostly well and going home. Nothing to worry about. Right?

Remember those capillaries that dilated in response to injury? Remember the slit pores that opened up and the fluid that poured out? Well, those slit pores are going to close up again, and when they do, all that fluid out in the periphery will get picked up and pulled back into the vascular space. If you are young and healthy you get rid of it when you urinate. If you are an old person with a bad heart and bad lungs, you hold onto it, become fluid overloaded, go into congestive heart failure, pulmonary edema, become hypoxic, have a lethal dysrhythmia, and die. Not exactly the outcome you were looking for.

What are the first two signs that a patient is going into congestive heart failure? (Before shortness of breath, before the numbers go bad.) Heart rate and respiratory rate begin to climb. The only way you see it is by looking at trends. The urine output is less than it had been before, but not necessarily abnormally low. By the time the patient has overt symptoms, the compensatory mechanisms have failed.

A lot of our post-op patients are sent home before this reabsorption – diuresis phase occurs. They come back into clinics and ERs, or are discharged into extended care facilities too soon and then go into failure. The very fact that the patient is still in the hospital should be a very big clue that the doctor expects this to happen to this patient. Watch them closely.

Compartment Syndrome

11

All the muscle bundles in your body are wrapped in fascia. The fascia is somewhat flexible. If you poke on your muscles it gives somewhat, but it does not expand indefinitely. Because of this, it has the characteristics of a fixed space. These compartments are distinct and non-communicating. Inside the compartments are muscle, nerve, and blood vessels.

To have good circulation in the muscle compartment, the blood needs to flow into the compartment, through the compartment, and out the other side. In order for this to occur, the pressure inside the compartment must never exceed the perfusion pressure. Should the pressure inside the compartment exceed the perfusion pressure, flow into the compartment will slow and stop. This is called compartment syndrome.

There are two main pathways to allow the pressure inside the compartment to exceed the perfusion pressure. The first one is for the pressure inside the compartment itself to go up—for example, if the patient bleeds into it. The pressure may also increase through intensive muscle use, burns, intra-arterial injections, decreased serum osmolality (i.e. nephritic syndrome), IVs infused into the compartment, venomization from snake bite, or "lying on limb." In a "lying on limb" situation, the patient is so debilitated from age, illness, alcohol, or drugs that he cannot arrange his limbs in such a way that there is good blood flow in the extremities. This is the drunk who passes out with his arm over the back of a chair or the elderly person who falls and stays in that position until help arrives to straighten her up and reestablish blood flow.

Anytime that you interrupt blood flow and reestablish it later, your patient is at risk for compartment syndrome. That would include any of your vascular surgery patients and many of your orthopedic patients, anyone who has been in shock, or anyone who has had a cardiac arrest. Also at risk are patients whose NBP cuffs pumped up, didn't go back down and no one noticed it for several hours.

The second pathway into compartment syndrome is to shrink the size of the compartment while all other factors remain the same. Casting does this beautifully. Every ER used to have a fully equipped cast room. You break it, we cast it. This is no longer true. Today you are told to take this nice splint and go home. Note the Velcro closures? Loosen them if it gets tight. Come back after the swelling is gone and we will give you a nice fiberglass cast in a color of your choice. We now do it this way because of compartment syndrome.

Other things that can shrink the size of the compartment are hematomas, infiltrated IVs, and burns, particularly ones that go all the way around the limb. So the two pathways into muscle compartment syndrome are to increase the pressure in the compartment or to shrink down the size of the compartment.

In compartment syndrome, for whatever reason, the pressure in the compartment exceeds the perfusion pressure. Because of this, blood flow into the compartment slows or stops, depending on the severity of the problem. Less oxygen is delivered to the tissues, they go anaerobic, and cannot generate the ATP they need. They become dysfunctional and begin excreting lactic acid as an end product of anaerobic metabolism. Things are not going well.

The body considers being anaerobic an injury and sets off inflammation—the response to injury. Out come the mediators, the capillaries dilate, their slit pores open up, out goes the fluid, which in turn increases the pressure in the compartment, thereby decreasing flow into it. And around and around we go in a cycle doomed to get worse. Lactic acid excreted into the muscles hurts, and it is supposed to. It is your body's way of saying, "Stop, stupid. We've gone anaerobic here!" If you stop or slow your exercise rate, the pain goes away as oxygen-laden blood makes it into the cells, restoring aerobic metabolism.

If insufficient oxygen is delivered to the cells, they can't make ATP the way they should, so they can't run their Na+ - K+ - ATP pumps the way they should. The cells swell up, become dysfunctional, and if it goes on long enough, the cells rupture, leaving tissue necrosis in its wake. And once the cells are gone, they *never* come back again. It is not a matter of sending the patient to PT to build the muscle back up again. It is permanently gone. A patient can lose his muscle bundle, his limb, and his life. A patient can die from compartment syndrome via metabolic acidosis and/or septic shock.

The most common place to see compartment syndrome is in the lower leg after high-velocity injuries. Possibly as many as 30% of all orthopedic cases get compartment syndrome. But remember, like everything else, compartment syndrome occurs on a continuum. You can have so little of it we hardly notice it, you can die from it, or experience any point in between these extremes.

If it is so devastating, how do you pick it up in the clinical setting? Over the years we have taught many ways to assess patients for compartment syndrome. We taught nurses to look for pain, paraesthesia, pallor, pilothermia (burning pain), and pulselessness. However, these signs depend on having a patient who can feel and talk coherently. You don't always get that.

So how do you tell? Assuming that your patient can feel, you tell with pain. Unrelenting pain that cannot be medicated to a tolerable level should alert you to the possibility of compartment syndrome. You should be able to medicate to a tolerable level (not gone, but tolerable) any and all post-op and trauma pain. If you can't, suspect compartment syndrome. Pain should get better every day, and if it is still at the same level day after day, get suspicious.

Patients who scream and cry no matter how much pain medication they are given, or ones who have to have Narcan to reverse the all the narcotics you have been giving them to make them comfortable, may be tying to tell you that they have an ischemic event going on. The pain from lactic acid buildup in muscles is extreme and unrelenting until adequate blood flow is restored. When the pain stops either the muscle bundle is dead or sufficient oxygen is now present for aerobic metabolism. There is a six hour window within which to restore oxygen delivery to the muscle bundle before it becomes necrotic – never to be revived.

If you suspect compartment syndrome, what are you going to do about it? First, if there is a cast on the extremity, get it cut off *now!* Do not hesitate! What if you cut a cast off and there isn't compartment syndrome present? Have you done a bad thing? No. Somebody puts a new cast on. Big deal. But what if compartment syndrome is present and you don't cut the cast off? Have you done something wrong? *Oh, yes.*

Remember: time is of the essence. Every minute results in more dead cells. You don't have time to page the doctor and wait around for a return call. Cut the cast off, then call the doctor and tell him what you did. You can't go wrong cutting a cast off. You can be very wrong in waiting. When you or someone who knows how cuts a cast off, remember to go all the way through the cast with the saw and down to the skin with your bandage scissors. Sometimes the wrap that is put on before the cast is the source of the stricture. By the same token, patients with only ace wraps on their extremities can have the same problems as casted patients. If the patient has unrelenting pain, remove the wrap.

If we determine that compartment syndrome is present, what are we going to do about it? The problem is one of excessive pressure in the compartment. How bad is it really? You can insert a needle into the compartment attached to a manometer and follow the pressure. Remember, we are again on a continuum—"awful" to "not so bad." If it's "not so bad," we can try the benign neglect approach (wait and see). If it is "awful," we need to act.

What is done is something called a fasciotomy. You literally fillet the extremity open down to the offending muscle bundle, slit the fascia to relieve the pressure in the bundle, and hopefully get enough perfusion going to stop the necrotic process. Fasciotomy in the past has meant cutting open the extremity and let nursing students do wet to dry dressing changes in the wound. Today we have the wound vac to aid the patient's healing, but you still start with a gaping wound.

In caring for these patients we return to the standard of oxygenation and perfusion. If this patient has an O_2 sat of 97% why does he need external oxygen? Because we are trying to effect oxygen delivery within the ischemic bundle and keep some $Na+ - K+ - ATP$ pumps

140

running. Keep the patient well-hydrated. Remember he is losing fluid into the bundle, and you need to keep perfusion pressures up. Those perfusion pressures are also aided by keeping the limb level with the body. This will give you the best mean arterial pressure (MAP) without increasing intra-compartmental pressure and therefore giving the best chance of blood flow into the bundle.

Complications of compartment syndrome are permanent nerve damage (the ones that move your hands and feet), loss of the limb, cosmetic deformity, infection and all its sequella down to SIRS, ARDS, and death on a ventilator. However, the sooner it is picked up the better the prognosis. For patients who cannot feel, you need to rely on you neuro-vascular checks—warmth of the extremity, capillary refill, pulse, etc. By the time you have lost the pulse, you've probably lost the game. Losing the pulse is a very late sign of compartment syndrome. Unrelenting pain is your best sign. Remember that pain should be better every single day, and if it isn't, that's not normal. Suspect compartment syndrome.

In the picture at right we see a patient who has had a good outcome from compartment syndrome, but look at the right leg. Would you like that leg? Muscle bundles are forever gone, making this leg permanently weaker than the other. There is terrible scaring with what appears to be skin grafts filling in between. And look at the rotation on the foot. This patient has foot drop. What a mess. We always assume that our patients don't have compartment syndrome. They really have to scream and carry on a lot to get our attention. Because compartment syndrome is *so* devastating, please, for all your patients who could potentially have it, assume that 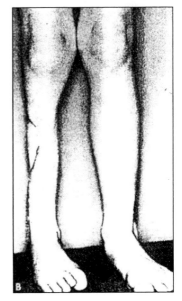 they *do* have it. Make them prove to you that they don't have it. If you have even the least suspicion that a patient might have compartment syndrome, get the cast cut off *immediately* and call a doctor.

GI Emergencies

12

G I emergencies come in three kinds: 1) hemorrhage, 2) mechanical obstruction causing ischemia, and 3) ischemia from venous and arterial constriction secondary to systemic shock. When you die, one hundred percent of the time you die from a lethal dysrhythmia. So, how can a GI bleed cause a lethal dysrhythmia? Easy. Remember the four things that must be balanced to keep the heart beating are:

- Normal pH
- Balanced electrolytes
- Oxygen
- Glucose

Hemorrhage to Lethal Dysrhythmia

$\downarrow$ volume $\rightarrow$ $\downarrow$ BP $\rightarrow$ $\downarrow$ oxygen delivery $\rightarrow$ anaerobic metabolism

$\rightarrow$ $\downarrow$ pH $\rightarrow$ lethal dysrythmia

also

$\downarrow$ O2 into the heart $\rightarrow$ $\downarrow$ repolarization of the action potential $\rightarrow$

lethal dysrythmia

There is less volume for circulation, so less oxygen is delivered to the cells. The cells go anaerobic, stop functioning properly, and begin cranking out lactic acid. Enough lactic acid changes the pH to a metabolic acidosis. That is one pathway into lethal dysrhythmia. Also, less oxygen is delivered into the heart, it can't make enough ATP to repolarize the action potential, and that is another pathway into lethal dysrhythmia. As you well know, someone having a GI emergency can die very quickly.

In the same way that plaque builds up in your heart, carotids, or legs, it can also build up in the mesenteric arteries. If this happens, flow decreases as does ATP production, function, and infrastructure repair. You can infarct the gut just like you can infarct anything else. If you don't take care of infrastructure repair you can perforate the gut—big or small—which can make you very septic, leading to SIRS, leading to ARDS, leading to death on a ventilator. You can destroy your liver causing death from hepatic failure with all that it entails.

You can also aspirate and have a terrible electrolyte imbalance. *Aspirate? Aspirate what? These patients aren't eating, what could they aspirate?* You and I produce eight liters of digestive fluids a day. We use it to digest our foods. It is very rich in electrolytes and used to make hydrochloric acid, bicarb, and pancreatic enzymes. As we digest our food and things move on through the gut, the water and electrolytes are picked up and recycled into the body. The problem occurs when an obstruction of some type keeps things from flowing on through. You continue making the digestive enzymes, but they don't make it down to the pick-up point, and the volume builds up like water behind a dam. This is what the patient aspirates and where the deficit in fluid and electrolytes occur. Remember, you don't have to actually be eating food to generate digestive juices, all you need do is *think* about it.

You can also have an ischemic gut from the vasoconstriction caused by systemic shock. This is a good time to look at the effects of shock. First, let's look at the cellular effects of shock. On a cellular level, what is occurring when insufficient oxygen is delivered to the cell?

Cellular Effects of Shock

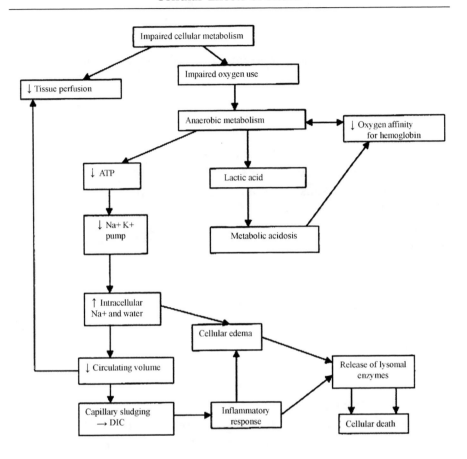

One definition of shock is that insufficient oxygen has been delivered to the cell to maintain aerobic metabolism. Because of this, the functions of the cell cannot be maintained, and the cell also begins to make lactic acid. Enough lactic acid in the system causes a metabolic acidosis to develop. As I said earlier, being alkalotic will cause the red blood cell to hang on to oxygen at a cellular level, but being acidic will keep it from attaching in the first place. Acidosis decreases the affinity of oxygen for hemoglobin, making our problem worse.

Now that the metabolism is anaerobic, there is insufficient ATP being generated, and the Na+ - K+ - ATP pumps are not working well. The cell begins to swell up with water, causing cellular edema and dysfunction. If this goes on long enough, the swelling will begin to pull lysomal membranes apart releasing caustic enzymes into the cell, producing cellular death. Enough dead cells and you get a dead human being.

Also, because there is so much of the body's water in the cells, there is a decrease in circulating volume. This decrease in volume causes changes in capillary flow via the pre- and post-capillary sphincters. The patient develops capillary sludging and goes into DIC. DIC is the hematological component of SIRS, setting off the inflammatory process through out the body, causing the destruction of lysomal membranes, and thereby cellular death. This is what is happening in every cell of the body as soon as insufficient oxygen is delivered to meet their metabolic needs.

GI BLEEDS

The problem with GI bleeds is that they cause you to lose volume and oxygen-carrying capacity. When making red blood cells—or anything else—problems of deficiency can have one of three causes: there is insufficient raw material available for building, the factory is not working right, or you are having a loss of the manufactured product.

Raw Material + Factory – Loss = Supply

Deficiencies in the supply of raw material (biological substrates)needed for manufacturing can occur because it was not eaten, absorbed in the gut, or transported to the factory. Problems in the manufacturing of substances can come from assembly lines producing too much, too little, or an inferior quality of the desired substance. Supply is also determined by how much of the product is being lost from or destroyed by the body. Some early artificial heart valves are known to destroy red blood cells and GI bleeds will cause them to be lost from the body.

Chronic GI bleeds are frequently detected because the patient develops an iron deficiency anemia. You recycle all of the iron used in your body to make red blood cells. When the body makes a new red blood cell it lasts about 120 days. Then it gets old and ratty, you tear it up, throw a lot of it away, but you recycle 100% of the iron back into the bone marrow to make new red blood cells. If a person develops an iron deficiency anemia, one easy way to make that happen is to have the red blood cells fall out of your body before the iron can be recycled. A slow, chronic GI bleed will do this nicely.

Let's look next at every nurse's favorite: the massive GI bleed.

Suppose a patient has just had a massive GI bleed. One of the first things you get is a propulsive movement of the gut-causing diarrhea. The effect of this is that the body doesn't have to metabolize all of that protein; the nurse can clean it up. The body considers this a plus. The patient is now volume-depleted. This triggers venous and arterial vasoconstriction. The venous constriction has the effect of increasing blood volume, and the arterial constriction increases perfusion pressures to help keep the blood circulating to vital areas. When you vasoconstrict into the skin it becomes cold, clammy, diaphoretic.

Vasoconstrict into the kidneys and they stop making urine. If you do not keep your kidneys flushed, they literally clog up with debris, causing acute tubular necrosis, renal failure, and death. Decreasing blood flow into the gut decreases function, repair, and peristalsis. You can infarct the mesenteric arteries and / or perforate the gut causing sepsis and SIRS, destroy the liver, and be dead from that.

Decreased blood flow into the heart is called myocardial ischemia. If you are inclined to feel it, it is called angina. The effect of it is decreased contractility leading to congestive heart failure, and you can have an MI. Also, with your change in level of consciousness from the hypovolemic event, you can have a stroke. The question becomes, "How in the world can you have an MI or a stroke from a hypovolemic event?" Easy.

Let's say a patient has some plaque in the carotid or left anterior descending artery in the heart. It may not be causing a problem, it may be at critical mass, or anything in between these two extremes.

Everything is just fine until the hypovolemic episode, when the blood flow is either cut off or so severely restricted that flow slows down, the vessel walls come closer together, and a clot forms, completing the MI or CVA.

147

The way you would prevent this from happening is to keep the walls of the blood vessel pushed apart. What could you use to do this? Fluid. Lots and lots of fluid. Preferably you should use normal saline as it stays within the vessel better than some of the others.

Conveying Your Concerns

13

These are statements written into patients' charts by people who were formerly thought to be intelligent.

- *The patient has chest pain if she lies on her side for over a year.*

- *On the second day the knee was better, on the third day it disappeared.*

- *She felt no rigors or shaking chills, but her husband states she was hot in bed last night.*

- *The patient is tearful and crying constantly. She also appears to be depressed.*

- *The patient has been depressed since she began seeing me in 1993.*

- *Discharge status: alive, but without permission.*

- *Healthy appearing, decrepit 69 year old male, mentally alert but forgetful.*

- *The patient refused autopsy.*

- *The patient had no previous history of suicide.*

- *The patient has left white blood cells at another hospital.*

- The patient's medical history has been remarkably insignificant with only a 40 pound weight gain in the last three days.

- The patient had waffles for breakfast and anorexia for lunch.

- Between you and me, we ought to be able to get this lady pregnant.

- Since she can't get pregnant with her husband, I thought you might like to work her up.

- She is numb from her toes down.

- While in the ER, she was examined, x-rated, and sent home.

- The skin was moist and dry.

- Occasional, constant, infrequent headaches.

- Patient alert and unresponsive.

- Rectal examination revealed a normal size thyroid.

- She stated that she had been constipated most of her life until she got a divorce.

- Both breasts were equal and reactive to light and accommodation.

- Examination of the genitalia reveals that he is circus sized.

- The patient was to have a bowel resection, however, he took a job as a stockbroker instead.

- Skin: somewhat pale but present.

- The pelvic exam will be done later on the floor.

- The patient was seen in consultation with Dr. Smith, who felt we should sit on the abdomen, and I agree.

- Large brown stool ambulating in the hall.

- The patient has two teenaged children, but no other abnormalities.

CONVEYING YOUR CONCERNS

Be organized in stating your case. Chronological order, complete vital signs, lab data. Say it all: who, what, when, where, what did you do, effect, what are you doing now, who did you tell, what did they say.

You have been a very diligent observer, and now you need to convey your concerns to other people. How do you get them to pay attention and see what you see? You must paint a vivid picture whether you are charting or doing a verbal report. To you, the event is in 3-D living color. To the doctor on the phone it can come across as flat, one-dimensional, in shades of grey. They have to see what you see. You must be organized in stating your case. Put everything in chronological order with complete vital signs and lab data. No skipping around, no late entries. The questions that need answering are: who, what, when, where.

Record what you did and what effect it had. We usually remember what we did, but tend to neglect recording effect of our actions. You gave him a nitroglycerine tablet for his chest pain? That's nice. How is he? Dead on the floor or sitting in the chair reading a book? You accidentally dc'd his epidural catheter so you started him on oral pain medication? How is he? Writhing in pain or watching the football game on TV?

What are you doing now? When you sign off your charting it looks like you never went into the patient's room again. Actually, you were in there a lot. You hung a new antibiotic, the doctor came by, RT gave a neb treatment for you—it was a busy place. But if you look at the charting, it looks like you said, *"Well, my shift is over. I hope he lives until they get out of report."* When you sign off your charting always say what you are continuing to do about the problem so that it shows your continued presence and attention to the patient.

Who did you tell and what did they say? You have a concern about this patient and the doctor does not share your concern. What do you do? Nurses frequently say, "I'm going to chart, chart, chart. He's going to be sorry he messed with me!" Or change "chart" to "call him back" and you have two strategies that do nothing to help the patient. If you have a disagreement with a doctor over treatment—or lack thereof— did you know that nurses are being held legally responsible for going up the chain of command? It is not something you get to do if you feel like it. You *must* go up the chain of command. In the good old days we could do it if we felt like it. today it is a legal requirement. If you don't go up the chain of command, and the doctor is sued, you will be sitting at the defendant's table with him.

Every medical *everything* has a medical head. Teaching hospitals use the resident-attending system. One of the functions of the medical head is to deal with your concerns about a patient's medical care. They would rather be awakened in the middle of the night than come in the next day and find out something untoward has happened to a patient that could have been prevented if you had gone up the chain of command.

Sometimes nurses are afraid to go up the chain of command for fear that they might be wrong. If you do activate the chain, and you were wrong, have you harmed the patient? No. What if you don't go up the chain of command and you where right. Have you harmed the patient? *Yes!* You must be prepared to occasionally be wrong, but most of the time you will be right. If you feel that strongly about something, you are usually right. Listen to your intuition.

Sometimes the doctor is very tuned in to what we are trying to explain, but we don't provide enough information on which to base a decision. We throw a bunch of numbers at them. Two patients can have the exact same vital signs with one getting better and one dying. You have to give the doctor some clues as to how the patient is doing with those numbers.

Vital information for the physician

- diaphoretic
- work effort
- fatigability
- patient's body position
- is the patient passing the look test,
- patient says this is the "worst ever",
- patient says this is "different from previous"
- any signs of poor cardiac output
- any signs of compartment syndrome
- new onset heart murmur

Is the patient diaphoretic? We now know that is a very ominous sign, signifying maximal sympathetic stimulation. How hard is the patient working to achieve those numbers? How long do you think he can keep it up? Fatigability can cause a sudden deterioration in a patient's condition.

What is the patient's body position? Is he lying flat in bed? Does he have the head of the bed up 30 degrees? Or is he like one patient I had who had pulled a chair over to the sink, put a pillow across the sink, and was trying to sleep with severe pulmonary edema. The patient's body position will tell you how stressed he is with those numbers.

If the patient has had this occur before, is this event the same as past ones? More or less severe? Episodes that are the "worst ever" or "different from previous" require a doctor. Remember, patients usually don't differentiate. You must ask, "Is this the usual and accustomed . . . ?" Is the patient passing the "Look Test"? Is the patient exhibiting any of the signs of poor cardiac output that were talked about earlier?

- Change in level of consciousness
- Respiratory distress anywhere on the continuum
- Heart rate up
- Liver down
- GI problems increased
- Urine output decreased
- Exercise capacity has dropped off

Is the girth increased or the amount of edema changing. This is more difficult to assess in the post-op patient because all post-op patients are edematous secondary to the capillary slit pores opening and fluid pouring out in the response to injury. Does the patient have any signs of compartment syndrome? Does the patient have a new onset heart murmur?

These are things the doctor has to know to make any kind of a rational decision about the patient. You have to paint a vivid picture for the doctor, and help the doctor see what you see.

PATIENT HISTORY

You've just done your physical assessment on a patient and you hear a heart murmur. How do you find out if he had the murmur yesterday? The easiest and most accurate way to find out is to look in the "Impression" section of the doctor's H&P. This is where the doctor lays it out clear as a bell what is wrong with this patient: aortic stenosis, atrial fibrillation, coumadin therapy, Type II diabetes, etc.

This information is worth its weight in gold, and it belongs on the patient's Kardex in the history section. Our patients complain over and over that we think we can come into their rooms and take care of them and we don't have a clue who they are. You might get away with it for a while, but the day will come when you will make a big mistake because you didn't know the patient's history. Our patients are sicker than ever before and our care must be more comprehensive than ever before.

An elderly lady had colon cancer and needed a colectomy. She also had a bad heart. The surgeon sent her to a cardiologist and said, "Do your best." The cardiologist took her off to the cath lab, angio-plastied several of her coronary arteries, started her on cardiac drugs, stabilized her, and set her back to the surgeon saying, "Good luck." She did very well post-op. She began to drink on time, eat on time, and was due to go home the next day when she crashed and burned during the middle of the night.

Her cardiac meds had never been restarted post-op. The history section on her Kardex was blank. None of the nurses taking care of her had any idea she had had an angioplasty done two weeks previous. Was it important for them to know? You bet it was, and by not know-ing they greatly compromised this patient's care. *"But, wait,"* you might say. *"It's not my job to start the meds back up!"* Have you figured out what your job as a nurse is yet? You are the great coordinator and sug-gester. It is the nurse that says to the doctor, *"Is it time to . . . ?"* Or *"Would you like to . . . ?"* When the nurse doesn't know the patient's history, care suffers.

What is caring anyway? What does it mean to care? The best def-inition I ever heard for the word caring came from holocaust survivor Elie Wiesel in his book *Night*. He said caring was having a willingness to intervene. If you care if your patient goes home again, one of the most powerful things you can do is to get the patient's history from the impression section of the H&P, put it on the patient's Kardex, and incor-porate it into your spiel for report. Your spiel goes something like: "Down in room 234 is Mr. Smith, who is a 67-year-old patient of Dr. Jones in with a thoracotomy, *and who has a history of . . . .*" This way, everyone sitting in report hears that the patient only has one kidney, or hears that this man has already had two sets of heart bypass grafts, or hears that the surgery was done for cancer. If you do this, you will greatly enhance the patient's care and increase his chances for survival. If you don't, you might get away with it, you might not. You can't be the patient's advocate if you don't know who the patient is.

Summary

S ubclinical signs proceed clinical signs. If I had to choose only one vital sign to follow, it wouldn't be blood pressure. It would be heart rate. Heart rate is a direct look into the patient's heart at stroke volume, and how much blood comes out with each beat. Heart rate goes up and down in response to volume (preload), contractility, metabolic demand, and work load (afterload). Increasing heart rate is the first indicator that patients are fluid overloaded, hypovolemic, infected, and hypoxic.

Because the heart and lungs are so closely tied together, when the heart rate begins to climb, the respiratory rate frequently begins to climb also. Respiratory rate beginning to climb is the first sign of respiratory distress. It is the first sign of patients going into congestive heart failure, ARDS, or other hypoxic events. It is compensation for metabolic acidosis—trying to blow off CO_2 and compensate for the lactic acidosis being produced on a cellular level. Patients becoming septic will show this early sign.

How long the subclinical sign lasts will vary from patient to patient. The younger and healthier they are when they enter their event, the longer they will be able to compensate. Some patients seem to crash and burn all at once, but if you go back into their vital signs, subclinical signs have been present for days and the patient had pretty good compensatory mechanisms that allowed him to hide overt symptoms from you. But the signs are there if you know what to look for—heart rate and respiratory rate starting to climb, and for the patient going into CHF, the urine output becomes less that it was before.

Our patients are sicker than ever, and there are fewer and fewer nurses involved in direct patient care. The nurse must look for trends in vital signs to see catastrophe coming. *Do not* rely on your nurse's aide to report abnormal vital signs. They are trained to *take* vital signs, not *interpret* them. It is the nurse who frequently stands between the patient and an emergency. Look for the subclinical signs of impending doom and prevent that crisis.

STUDY PACKAGE
CONTINUING EDUCATION
CREDIT INFORMATION

CRISIS PREVENTION:
SUBCLINICAL SIGNS OF IMPENDING DOOM

Thank you for choosing PESI Healthcare as your continuing education provider. Our goal is to provide you with current, accurate and practical information from the most experienced and knowledgeable speakers and authors.

Listed below are the continuing education credit(s) currently available for this self-study package. **Please note, your state licensing board dictates whether self study is an acceptable form of continuing education. Please refer to your state rules and regulations.*

Nurses: PESI HealthCare, LLC, Eau Claire is an approved provider of continuing nursing education by the Wisconsin Nurses Association Continuing Education Approval Program Committee, an accredited approver by the American Nurses Credentialing Center's Commission on Accreditation. This approval is accepted and/or recognized by all state nurses associations that adhere to the ANA criteria for accreditation. This learner directed educational activity qualifies for **3.6 contact hours**. PESI Healthcare certification: CA #06538

Procedures: 1. Read book.
2. Complete the post-test/evaluation form and mail it along with payment (if necessary) to the address on the form.

Your completed test/evaluation will be graded. If you receive a passing score (80% and above), you will be mailed a certificate of successful completion with earned continuing education credits. If you do not pass the post-test, you will be sent a letter indicating areas of deficiency, references to the appropriate sections of the manual for review and your post-test. The post-test must be resubmitted and receive a passing grade before credit can be awarded.

If you have any questions, please feel free to contact our customer service department at 1-800-843-7763.

PESI HealthCare, LLC
200 SPRING ST. STE B, P.O. BOX 1000
EAU CLAIRE, WI 54702-1000

Product Number: ZHS009740   **CE Release Date:** 4/11/05

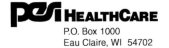
PESI HealthCare
P.O. Box 1000
Eau Claire, WI 54702
(800) 843-7763

Crisis Prevention:
Subclinical Signs of
Impending Doom
ZNT009740

This home study package includes CONTINUING
EDUCATION FOR ONE PERSON: complete & return this
original post/test evaluation form.

ADDITIONAL PERSONS interested in receiving credit
may photocopy this form, complete and return with a
payment of $25.00 per person CE fee. A certificate of
successful completion will be mailed to you.

For office use only
Rcvd. _____
Graded _____
Cert. mld. _____

C.E. Fee: **$25**   Credit card # _____

Exp. Date _____

Signature _____

V-Code* _____ (*MC/VISA/Discover: last 3-digit # on signature
panel on back of card.) (*American Express: 4-digit # above account # on face
of card.)

Mail to: PESI HealthCare, PO Box 1000, Eau Claire, WI 54702, or
Fax to: PESI HealthCare (800) 675-5026 (fax all pages)

Name (please print): _____ _____ _____
                              LAST   FIRST   M.I.

Address: _____

City: _____ State: _____ Zip: _____

Daytime Phone: _____

Signature: _____

• Date you completed this Independent Study Package: _____

• Actual time (# of hours) taken to complete this offering: _____ hours

RESOURCE

Please circle your responses, rating and overall impressions of this book.

	Excellent				Poor
Content	5	4	3	2	1
Presentation of Material	5	4	3	2	1
Knowledge and Expertise	5	4	3	2	1

Comments _____

_____

_____

_____

LEARNING OBJECTIVES

Please evaluate this book's effectiveness in communicating the following objectives:

	Excellent				Poor
Identifying the difference in clinical vs. sub-clinical signs and the body's compensatory mechanisms for homeostasis.	5	4	3	2	1
Describing how all the organ systems are totally interrelated and interdependent.	5	4	3	2	1
Determining how to pull signs and symptoms into the big picture, rather than letting them stand alone.	5	4	3	2	1
Utilizing the critical thinking model to see the multiple dimensions in clinical situations.	5	4	3	2	1
Explaining how to convey concerns about a patient to physicians on the phone, in shift reports, and in charting.	5	4	3	2	1

POST-TEST QUESTIONS

1. What is the only power source for the human body?

    a. PAF

    b. ATP

    c. AS

    d. TNF

2. Which of the following is NOT occurring in the heart during diastole?

    a. filling

    b. repolarization

    c. ventricular contraction

    d. coronary perfusion

3. Cardiac output is a factor of:

    a. heart rate and stroke volume

    b. heart rate and respiratory rate

    c. heart rate and basal metabolic rate

    d. heart rate and circadian rate

4. Rales can be heard in the lungs of patients with:

    a. right heart failure

    b. left heart failure

    c. hypovolemia

    d. increased contractility

5. Edema is a good indication of a post-op patient's fluid status?

    a. True

    b. False

For additional forms and information on other PESI products, contact:
**Customer Service; PESI HEALTHCARE; P.O. Box 1000; Eau Claire, WI 54702
(Toll Free, 7 a.m.-5 p.m. central time, 800-843-7763).
www.pesihealthcare.com**

**Thank you for your comments.
We strive for excellence and we value your opinion.**

Professional Resources Available from PESI HealthCare

Resources for Mental Health Professionals

Addiction, Progression & Recovery, by Dale Kesten, LCSW, LADC

Assessing and Treating Trauma and PTSD, by Linda Schupp, Ph.D

Borderline Personality Disorder—Struggling, Understanding, Succeeding, by Colleen E. Warner, Psy.D

Case Management Handbook for Clinicians, by Rand L. Kannenberg, MA

Clinicians Update on the Treatment and Management of Anxiety Disorders, by Deborah Antai-Otong, MS, RN, CNS, NP, CS, FAAN

Collaborative Healing: A Shorter Therapy Approach for Survivors of Sexual Abuse, by Mark Hirschfeld, LCSW-C, BCD & Jill B. Cody, MA

Delirium–The Mistaken Confusion, by Debra Cason-McNeeley, MSN, RNCS

Depression and Other Mood Disorders, by Deborah Antai-Otong, MS, RN, CNS, NP, CS, FAAN

Effective Strategies for Helping Couples and Families, by John S. Carpenter

Grief: Normal, Complicated, Traumatic, by Linda Schupp, Ph.D

Psychiatric Emergencies, by Deborah Antai-Otong, MS, RN, CNS, NP, CS, FAAN

Sociotherapy for Sociopaths: Resocial Group, by Rand L. Kannenberg, MA

Resources for Nurses & Other Healthcare Professionals

Heart and Lung Sounds Reference Library (Audio CD), by Diane Wrigley, PA-C

Infection Control and Emerging Infectious Diseases, by William Barry Inman

Legal and Ethical Standards for Nurses, by Sheryl Feutz-Harter

Managing Urinary Incontinence (Audio CD), by Carol Ann White, RN, MS, ANPC, GNPC

Mechanisms and Treatment of Disease: Pathophysiology—A Plain English Approach, by Mikel A. Rothenberg, MD

Oral Medication and Insulin Therapies: A Practical Guide for Reaching Diabetes Target Goals, by Charlene Freeman

Subclinical Signs of Impending Doom (Audio CD), by Carol Whiteside, RN, PhD(c)

Understanding X-Rays–A Plain English Approach, by Mikel A. Rothenberg

To order these or other PESI HealthCare products or to receive information about our national seminars, please call 800-843-7763

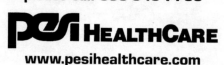

www.pesihealthcare.com